THE ⊕RIGINS ⊕F
PSYCHIC
PHEN⊕MENA

ALSO BY STAN GOOCH

The Dream Culture of the Neanderthals

Four Years On

Total Man

Personality and Evolution

The Neanderthal Question

The Paranormal

The Double Helix of the Mind

The Secret Life of Humans

THE ⊕RIGINS ⊕F PSYCHIC PHEN⊕MENA

POLTERGEISTS, INCUBI, SUCCUBI, AND THE UNCONSCIOUS MIND

STAN GOOCH

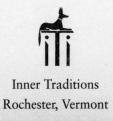

Inner Traditions

Rochester, Vermont

Inner Traditions
One Park Street
Rochester, Vermont 05767

ISBN-13: 978-1-59477-164-4 (pbk.)

Text design and layout by Jon Desautels

Printed in the United States

For Ezra Kogan

and

David Sawyer

C⊕NTENTS

PART THREE
INTENTIONS

We live in a truly dark age, lit only here and there by a few candles.

MARTYN PRYER

But the skeptics are happier in their singleness and their simplicity, happy that they do not, will not, realize the monstrous things that lie only just beneath the surface of our cracking civilization.

MONTAGUE SUMMERS

INTR⊕DUCTI⊕N

The hero of this book is a former police detective sergeant, now a bus driver. His testimony determined me to write it. He wrote to tell me that he was being visited nocturnally by various incubi and a succubus. A succubus is defined by the *Oxford Dictionary* as a female demon who makes love to men during the hours of darkness. An incubus is a demon who bears down upon people during their sleep, choking and suffocating them, but who also performs the sex act with women.

The significant point about his letter, the synchronistic point perhaps, was that I myself had recently begun receiving visits from a succubus.

Then, only a short time later, a well-known actress wrote to me asking for help. When I visited her she told me she had recently been attacked at night by an entity, an experience which had left her, apart from fearful, with a mouthful of dried blood. Two very interesting facts to emerge about her are that she is left-handed and has an extra nipple. These, of course, are the traditional marks of the medieval witch.

Other material came rapidly to hand. The film *The Entity,* for example, is based on an actual case reported by a psychiatrist. Here a woman was raped on several occasions by an entity or force, which left her with severe bruising and a damaged mind. In Italy, in 1983, a Scottish girl, Carol Compton, was denounced and tried as a witch. Objects are said to have moved in her presence without being touched, and in particular she was accused of starting three fires paranormally, when she herself was not physically present, in a child's bedroom.

The question of paranormal fire leads on to a recent case of what is called spontaneous human combustion. According to a Chicago police report, a woman burst spontaneously into flames while walking down a city street, in full view of many witnesses. Incidentally, the bizarre and so far inexplicable occurrence of human beings bursting into flames, in which the flesh of the victim is totally consumed while adjacent objects and sometimes even the victim's clothing remain unharmed, is one that otherwise skeptical scientists accept as factual. They have to. How can they reject the findings of coroners' inquests?

The surge of paranormal visitations described in this book is perhaps remarkable for its occurrence at a time when orthodox science has never been stronger, when Western academic opinion in general has never been more ready to pour scorn on what it considers to be the superstitious hysteria of fools. Yet, as this book shows, a growing number of doctors, scientists, and psychiatrists around the world are quietly reporting on aspects of the phenomena under discussion. Increasingly, too, their reports are appearing in the orthodox medical and scientific press.

The investigation of the remarkable events of a succubus–incubus visitation—and of such other allied phenomena as poltergeist attacks—leads us in fact not into some cuckooland of human gullibility and credulity, but into a still more remarkable and altogether real area, the human unconscious mind. In the professional literature we find much relevant documentation not only from "historical" sources such as Sigmund Freud, C. G. Jung, and their associates, but from modern, practicing psychiatrists like Morton Schatzman, Mary Williams, Lorna Selfe, Hervey Cleckley, R. L. Moody, and many others. We find, for instance, a poltergeist–incubus attack occurring in a doctor's consulting room, a woman whose hallucinations became visible to others, and cases of multiple personality where the alternative, displacing personae exhibit not simply psychological characteristics different from those of the "real" occupant of the body but also different brain waves and other autonomic physiological responses. By no criteria whatsoever can we consider these alternative, usurping personae to be any less actual, any less genuine than the "normal" owner of consciousness—that is, than the "real" you who sits reading this book. So what, then, really is a human personality, and what are not so much the *limits* of its powers, as the full, unrealized *extent* of them? The answers to these questions prove to be far more daunting than any alleged world of spirits (the "explanation" usually put forward by occultists and paranormalists); they are so daunting, in fact, that the implications of the wholly authentic instances detailed here are currently totally excluded from "informed" modern Western consciousness. We shall as a passing exercise be documenting a deliberate (although perhaps not fully conscious) policy of total nondiscussion of these matters by mainstream Western academic psychology and psychiatry in particular and by Western science in general.

Is it the growing acceptance of supernormal phenomena by the public at large that is leading both to a renaissance of these dramatic events and, above all, to a willingness to stand up and be counted? Or is it the denial and repression by mainstream academic opinion of the forces involved (whatever they may prove to be) which increases the strength of those forces, so that what might otherwise be controlled and channeled bursts out in uncontrolled violence?

The point has certainly been reached where the phenomena in question must be made fully public. As the one-time detective sergeant put it: "This area doesn't just need investigating. It needs a bloody great searchlight."

I hope this book is his bloody great searchlight.

PART ONE

BEGINNINGS

INCUBI AND SUCCUBI
IN SUBURBIA

In the spring of 1981 Martyn Pryer, a former detective sergeant with the Metropolitan Police, wrote to tell me of some of his experiences with alternative reality. Of these, his experiences with apparently discarnate entities or demons are the most exciting, since they seem to go well beyond any form of "mere" hallucination. Martyn Pryer's own written accounts can hardly be bettered, and excerpts from these now follow.

Some aspects of Martyn's earlier life are more relevant to subsequent chapters. All that need be demonstrated here is that, while successfully pursuing a "straight" career, there had always been another more poetic side to Martyn's nature that prevented him from integrating finally with those (the majority of people) who go through life in a state of, as he puts it, "uncontrolled folly."

At the age of about four or five, after being put to bed, I would get up and sit on the windowsill, watching the sun set over the woods and fields at the back of the house. These moments are among the dearest memories of my childhood. . . .

By the age of eighteen I had become a fully fledged nature mystic. I used to wander in the woods and talk to the trees. I seemed to be floating as I wandered about late at night. I smelled the air and held my hands up to the rain. I allowed myself to merge with nature. It all sounds a bit daft when put into writing, but these were beautiful experiences. You are no doubt familiar with these kinds of accounts—but truly, words cannot describe them accurately.

Yet Martyn was no effete misfit. He was, for instance, already playing in his school's first rugby XV at the age of fourteen.

The first incident of direct interest occurred when Martyn was twenty-six. He was by then a detective sergeant in the Special Branch and assigned to port duty at Dover. He had taken digs in a small, old cottage outside the town. One night, having gone to bed, he found he could not sleep.

I gradually became aware of a "presence" in the room. This presence was very hostile. I put on the light, but there was nothing to be seen or heard. I put out the light again, but the presence was still there. To cut a long story short, I eventually fell asleep with the light on, and my police truncheon clutched in my hand. The next and subsequent nights were uneventful. The presence had gone. I now questioned my landlady circumspectly about the house. She told me that years previously, during the Second World War, the house had been troubled for a while by a ghost, and that one evening she had seen an old person's wrinkled face at the window of her kitchen. Around the same time she had once heard footsteps on the stairs.

This was an isolated incident in a period when Martyn had abandoned his beloved study of all forms of philosophy—when still a uniformed constable he had been known as "the Prof" by his colleagues—and had immersed himself in the technicalities of his Special Branch career, in marriage, in buying a house, and in starting a family. His two daughters became very involved in ballet classes, and he himself learned to play the piano. He smilingly describes his life from the age of twenty-four to thirty-five as "dreadfully suburban."

He then became increasingly depressed with the life of a detective sergeant, of working with colleagues whose only interests in life seemed to involve promotion and material possessions. As his unhappiness increased he finally sought and obtained a discharge from the force. He then spent two and a half years as a social worker and was at that point seconded to study for a formal qualification. This enterprise he abandoned after a year, and he went on to work for a time as a personnel officer in a security firm. Finally he became a bus driver, a job he has held ever since, which he finds has given him back his peace of mind and the freedom to think his own thoughts.

It was during his time as a social worker that Martyn rediscovered his beloved philosophy. He began reading everything he could lay his hands on concerning the human condition, the "how" and the "why" of human existence. In particular he began reading esoteric and paranormal texts.

Early in 1980, at the age of forty-one, Martyn began to undertake a personal investigation of alternative phenomena. He decided to experiment with hypnagogic imagery.

Hypnagogic imagery is experienced by many people just before they drop off to sleep. Flashes of imaginary scenes and incidents pass briefly before their eyes. With practice, it is possible to avoid falling asleep, at least for a time. Then the images become more vivid and semi-continuous. Their vividness and precise detail can, in fact, be remarkable. It was with this state, then, that Martyn began experimenting.

On going to bed I would place a folded handkerchief over my eyes to keep out any residual light, and then physically relax. I would allow myself to drift down towards sleep and then try to hold myself just barely awake.

During the next few months I would often wake at night bathed in sweat. I talked in my sleep, something I had never done before, and, once, during a vivid dream, I made an eerie high-pitched whining. I was aware that I was doing it, but knew I could not stop till the dream was over. All in all, I was now so restless a sleeper that my wife often went downstairs to sleep on the settee.

After some three weeks of attempting hypnagogy, and while still awake, I began to hear knocks, sometimes regularly spaced, one—two—three, and also less determinate thumps. These were quite different from house-settling noises or water pipes.

Martyn's experiments continued. He sometimes heard conversations going on around him. Once a male voice addressed him, to which he replied, and on another occasion a nasty female voice cackled in his ear.

As well as practicing hypnagogy he tried exercises he had read about for inducing out-of-the-body experiences and also attempted the kundalini effect—an exercise where one tries to cause unconscious energies to flow up through the spine[1]—with varying results. Then:

One night, while relaxing and hypnagoging, I experienced a pressure on my toes. Shortly afterwards I felt a distinct tug on the hair on the right side of my head. It was a strong tug, quite distinct, but not painful. I was lying on my back at the time with my head on the pillow.

A few nights later I had my first seizing experience. I had turned on my side to sleep, and was in fact approaching sleep. With a massive "whoosh," which I heard quite clearly, I was seized from behind by a man-like entity. It pinioned my legs with its legs, and my arms with its arms, and began breathing heavily in my ear. I was fully conscious, but could not move a muscle. The psychological impact of this event was shattering, totally outside any previous experience I had had. I had no explanations to fall back on—indeed, I was too panic-stricken to contemplate any analytical ideas. I nevertheless felt this creature to be primitive, wanton, unprincipled, uncivilized—the opposite of all that is normally regarded as noble and good. A fiend had got me. It was Satan on my back.

Somehow a visionary experience now became entwined in the situation. I knew that I was still in bed (though that knowledge was very remote), but I was also standing in a very dark room—and in

full possession of my normal mental faculties. I knew that there
was a light switch just outside the room, and I managed to stagger
across the room with the "thing" clinging like a limpet to my back.
I managed to free my left arm. I reached through the doorway for
the light switch, only to find that this was hidden under a mass of
trailing wires and cables. Scrabbling around through the wires I
finally got to the switch. But before I could press it, as I was about
to do, I was released. I did not wake up. I had been awake all the
time. But with a "pop" the scene around me changed from the dark
room to my bedroom.

I cannot emphasize enough that this experience had a reality
beyond belief. I was there, "it" was there and "it" was real. Real,
solid and alive. It felt hostile and unbelievably alien, as though it
had indeed sprung from the "halls of Hell."

I don't mind admitting that this experience badly scared me.
Yet I was determined to go forward, not back.

There is a great deal to be said about many aspects of Martyn Pryer's
experiences. The seizing from behind and clinging on, not touching the
ground, very much recalls the "Old Man of the Sea" described in legends, for example. However, for the moment we continue to narrate
Martyn's further adventures.

A few nights later I was again seized. This time I was still on my
back practising hypnagogy, when I was suddenly possessed within
in a sudden "zap." There was no man-like entity. I was just held
"internally," unable to move a muscle, although I still had my full
conscious awareness. For a short time nothing further happened.
Then a great weight started to press down on me, all along the
length and width of my body. It grew heavier and heavier. I knew
distinctly that I was in my own bed and that it was not possible
for there to be a weight or anything else above me on the bed. Yet
here it was pressing down on me with ever increasing force. The
experience was horrifying. Suddenly I felt that this was enough and

that I must escape. It took a great effort on my part, an effort summoned up by sheer desperation. Then the thing was gone, leaving me very disturbed. [What Martyn was experiencing here was the traditional incubus rather than the succubus.] A couple of nights later I had turned over and was already asleep when I was again seized, again the internal seizure, not the external one. The seizure jolted me fully awake. I was again totally paralysed. This time I reacted immediately. I screamed mentally, "Get off, you bastard, get off" several times. And then it suddenly went. I now went back to sleep, this time more angry than frightened. Twice more that night I was seized—taken over, occupied. These were comparatively minor attacks, however, which I easily threw off.

Martyn had also begun to have many visionary experiences, in three dimensions, full color, touch, and sound, and once he sleepwalked in a rather unusual way. Then:

One night, having hypnagoged for a while, and then turned over on my side prior to going to sleep, I found myself suddenly in total darkness. I was fully awake and conscious—but I sensed that I was somehow in a different room. In "imagination" (a totally inadequate word to describe the reality of these experiences) I made my way over to where I sensed there was a window. Outside was a girl—she had been older than myself—whom I had once courted in my youth. I asked: "What are you doing here, Christine?" She replied: "You sent for me." I reached out and felt her face. I could really feel it. It was solid to my touch.

Then, zap, I was seized from behind. I was now fully awake, and fully aware of lying in my own bed in my own room, on my right side.

The entity which was clasping me from behind was not only anthropomorphic, but distinctly female. The effect of this realization was shattering—if I knew of any stronger word I would use it. The entity was rapacious. It moulded itself to my back and nuzzled the left side of the back of my neck. I was completely paralysed and could not even blink. Yet my own identity and will remained intact, and I was fully conscious.

Being now in a sense more used to these strange events—though still none the less completely amazed by them—I decided to wait and see what would happen. It seemed to me that the entity was displaying an intention—a desire that was entirely its own, and a kind of nasty intelligence. It seemed, obviously, to want to make love to me, in a crude and violent manner, although it was of course in the wrong position for actual copulation. We lay there together for a while, but the creature did little else. Gradually its presence faded, but right up to the last the pressure on my buttocks was almost painful, as though two huge hands were gripping me. Finally the effect was gone, and eventually I fell asleep.

We turn now to the experiences of the actress, Miss S. T., whom we shall call Sandy.

Sandy's early background is briefly as follows. At the age of two and a half she was involved in a serious car accident that left her face badly scarred. Plastic surgery is inappropriate in such cases until adolescence, when the face has ceased to grow. This facial scarring was one of the factors which caused Sandy to feel apart from other children—and for them in turn to reject her. As Alfred Adler demonstrated, such "organ inferiority" can be a powerful influence on the individual's behavior and the development of the personality. In addition, however, Sandy had three nipples and was left handed. She also suffered from dyslexia and could not read or write until the age of nine.

During childhood she sought comfort from the rejection of her schoolmates by spending much time in bed in conversation with two teddy-bears and an invisible figure whom she thought of mainly as Jesus. This figure spoke to her "in her head," and to it she addressed all her requests.

Many children have vivid relationships with toys and imaginary magical figures, but Sandy's lasted longer than most. There are also some grounds for regarding her imaginary companions as "familiars," since Sandy often wished she was a witch, so that she could take revenge on her schoolmates. At some point, too, in her childhood Sandy must also have understood the alleged significance of having three nipples—one of the most noted signs of the medieval witch. The devil was said to suck milk from such supernumerary nipples and indeed to have caused them to be there for this purpose. (Finally as an adult, Sandy discovered that she did indeed have some sort of ability to make absent people who had offended her unhappy during occasions when they should have been enjoying themselves.)

Nevertheless, as a youngster, apart from talking to imaginary figures, Sandy had no specific experiences that we could describe as paranormal or psychologically inexplicable. And in fact Sandy, like Martyn Pryer, was outstanding at sport and dancing—a kind of "closet extrovert." (Ultimately, she ran for her county.)

With the arrival of puberty (and some subsequent plastic surgery) Sandy, the "ugly duckling," was transformed into an unusually attractive woman—and one who was by now an academically high achiever. The tables had been completely turned. Sandy now had all the advantages over her female companions and male society in her pocket. In due course she became a successful actress, a member for a time of the Royal Shakespeare Company.

In her late twenties she had become fairly seriously interested in the intuitive-occult side of life and had frequently sought the advice of a professional psychic, Aleph. A few months prior to the incident described below, Sandy had played in a production of the Scottish play by Shakespeare (the name of which must not be mentioned in the theater) as one of the three witches. It is worth emphasizing here the very high level of superstition prevailing in theatrical circles. No doubt this dramatic role re-aroused Sandy's own view of herself as a witch. Then Aleph began warning Sandy that something rather evil was near her.

As a preface to Sandy's experience, one of Martyn Pryer's reports is relevant, in view of the parallels involved. The incident occurred some weeks before Martyn's first seizing experience. While practicing hypnagogy one night, Martyn saw a large, single eye, set in about an inch of flesh, staring at him. He thought it seemed to be feminine. For three weeks, each night, he and the eye stared at each other, without anything further happening. Now on this final night he grew angry with the "persecution." He snatched the handkerchief off his eyes and sat up in bed. The eye was still there, floating in space, up near the ceiling. He became yet more angry and willed the vision to fade. Gradually it did so, never to return.

Sandy had gone to bed, relaxed and rather cheerful, and slept easily. During the night she woke from dreamless sleep and looked around her in the darkness. The spotlamp in the corner of the ceiling had become a human eye, staring at her. Now she began to feel a pressure bearing down on her as she lay in bed. It was, she says, like a lover lying on top of her, making gentle rhythmic motions. (When I asked her if she was sure if this encounter had really been sexual, she replied: "Oh, I knew where the main pressure was, all right, don't worry.") At first she was not unduly disturbed by these strange events. One part of her was quite willing for the love-making to proceed, but another part of her knew that she wanted it to stop. The pressure suddenly increased dramatically and became painful. She began to struggle. Now a visionary element entered into the experience. She found herself being forced down through the mattress. Not only was there the crushing weight on top of her, but something else—a force—had seized her from behind and was dragging her down. She felt this other presence to be extremely evil and threatening and knew she must now resist. She managed (in her vision) to put a hand back up through the slats and the broken mattress and made a great effort to haul herself free. Suddenly the forces were gone. Extremely disturbed, she now got out of her bed and went into the bathroom to look at herself. Her mouth was rimmed with dark streaks of dried blood. When she opened her mouth it was full of black blood. An inspection revealed no sign of a nosebleed or any injury to her mouth or throat.

The next day Aleph instructed Sandy to wear a snake charm for protection; since then there has been no recurrence of the incident.

Perhaps the last word here should rest with Martyn Pryer. From a television program, he subsequently discovered that in the church of Hertogenbosh, the home town of the painter Hieronymous Bosch, high in the vaulted ceiling, is painted a huge single eye, set in about an inch of flesh.

My experiences with my own succubus have been, by contrast, extremely pleasant. But I never found my encounters with the supernormal, across half a lifetime, anything other than exciting and fascinating, never fearful. The succubus experience was nevertheless totally unexpected and quite different from anything else I had ever experienced.

I subsequently recalled that I had had one experience, in my midtwenties when developing as a trance medium, that could perhaps be seen as a forerunner. I was in bed on a Saturday morning, fully awake, but with eyes closed and quite unwilling to get up after the working week. The curtains were closed, but I was aware behind my closed eyes of the daylight percolating in. Then I felt a pressure and movement on the pillow next to my head. It was precisely the effect one has when someone else's hand presses down on a pillow on which one's head is resting. I was immediately alert, and rather thrilled, but I did not open my eyes. The "hand" continued to press down gently on the pillow. The movement was quite unmistakable. After a little while it stopped and I cautiously opened my eyes. There was nothing to be seen.

No such similar experience was to occur for the next twenty years. Then, I was once again lying in a bed in the early morning, awake but drowsy, with daylight already broken. I was waiting to slip for an hour or so into one or other of the areas of the alternative universe (see chapter 16), as I often do in the early mornings, when, with a strong sense of disbelief, I became aware of another person in bed with me. For a moment I totally dismissed the idea. Then she—it was a she—moved a little closer, pressing against me more urgently.

As Martyn Pryer says, one tries not to use vivid language in the telling of these matters for fear of sounding unconvincing. However, with a sense of rising excitement, which I tried to control (for it does not aid any phenomenon to "lose one's cool"), I realized that this was certainly my most profound paranormal experience to date, among many remarkable events.

I somehow knew that this was a "psychic entity." I knew it was not a real person who had got into my room by normal means. I tried to let the entity go on controlling the situation, but my own interest was naturally very intense. Without opening my eyes, I realized that the "person" in bed with me—in *front* of me, I should stress—was a composite of various girls I had once known (Martyn Pryer agrees on this point) including my ex-wife, but with other elements not drawn from my memories in any sense. In short, this entity, though possessing physical and even psychological attributes familiar to me, was nonetheless essentially its own independent self. It was not solely compounded of my imagination—or, at least, not entirely of elements which I consciously recognized. It was its own creature but seemed, as it were, to be using part of my own experience in order to present itself to me.

On this first occasion my conscious interest in the situation got the better of me, and the succubus gradually faded away. On subsequent occasions, however, the presence of the entity was maintained, until finally we actually made love.

I am as unwilling to go into the intimate details of the love making itself as I would be about those of any girl with whom I was having a relationship. I can only say that the experience is totally satisfying—a comment endorsed by Ruth's experience with her incubus–husband, described in chapter 10, and indeed by Carlotta in chapter 2. From some points of view the sex is actually more satisfying than that with a real woman, because in the paranormal encounter archetypal elements are both involved and invoked, a rare event in normal everyday relationships. For my own part, like the heroes of many folktales and fairy stories, I am more than happy to settle for a relationship with a succubus, and the world of real women (but what does "real" mean?) can go whistle. It is, I must add, perfectly possible to have a lifetime relationship with a succubus, thus: "for forty years Benedict of Berne had kept up amatory commerce with a succubus called Hermeline" (C. K. Sharpe, Law's Memoriall's 1818).

The psychological and physiological mechanics of what is going on in these experiences of Martyn, of Sandy, of Ruth, of Carlotta, and of mine and others is something we shall be considering in the rest of this book. For the moment, and referring specifically to my own case, I would say that the sense of touch is one hundred percent engaged. My remaining senses are somewhat less than one hundred percent engaged—and since I do not open my eyes, the normal vision is therefore totally excluded (although I sometimes see an "inward vision" of the visitor). Ruth, however, sees her incubus–husband perfectly clearly with her eyes fully open (chapter 10) and so does Carlotta (chapter 2). I am probably about five percent "dissociated" (to use the technical term) during my experiences: that is to say, I am about ninety-five percent awake and alert. I know what is happening. I know who I am and where I am. I am on a double mattress, on top of another double mattress, on the floor of the sparsely furnished attic flat where I sleep. I am also in another world that science does not recognize, but which mankind from the earliest times nevertheless knows well.

We have probably already seen enough in this book to realize that there is, after all, some kind of genuine basis to at least a proportion of the "fanciful superstitions" entertained in medieval and still earlier times. Are traditional "witch marks" sometimes the external sign of strange gifts, and is the "hovering single eye" an archetypal herald of strange visitations? (This phenomenon, of course, recalls the inner or "third eye" of mysticism, frequently discussed in esoteric texts.) What further phenomena in ancient accounts may the modern world also be forced to come to terms with?

It is quite clearly the case that the modern Western world view or universe view cannot as it stands incorporate even the phenomena so far discussed. On the contrary, the modern world seeks to deny them totally. As Martyn Pryer, Mrs. W. D. (see chapter 16), and others have remarked bitterly, there is no person in the Western academic or scientific establishment to whom one can turn for help or enlightenment in matters of this kind.

For my part, though I considered myself enlightened, until recently I still smiled when I heard, for instance, stories of "visible thought forms" allegedly produced by Tibetan mystics and others. These "creatures" are said to be able to move about independently of their creator and also to be visible and tangible to others. (Carlos Castaneda, as many will recall, has written of these matters in his Don Juan books.)

I no longer smile at such stories. My own feeling, now, is that there may literally be no limit to what can be achieved by the human subjective mind manipulating and actualizing itself in the external, objective universe around it.

2
DEMONS PAST AND ENTITIES PRESENT

Visitations of incubi, demons, entities, and other unknown forces are common in our own time, as the previous chapter has already begun to demonstrate. They are far commoner, in fact, than many people realize. Emphatically, these visitations do not happen in out-of-the-way places to people whose honesty, or at least whose intelligence, is questionable. They occur in modern Western cities, and they befall normal, articulate, highly intelligent individuals. Nor do they happen just at night, but also in broad daylight, sometimes in the presence of independent witnesses of standing. These visitations seem to be on the increase.

This book concentrates on the present day, even the present minute. There are, certainly, those—mystics, occultists, or whoever—who seem to prefer to have their phenomena taking place in the distant past. This circumstance may make such events seem more thrilling (although here they are in principle wrong—there is nothing more thrilling, in the right circumstances, than strange happenings in your own time). The location of phenomena in the distant past, certainly, allows the imagination to riot unchecked. Is perhaps the attraction of distant phenomena that they cannot be disproved? A sarcastic point, certainly, but possibly a true one.

But if phenomena only apparently occurred in the past but now no longer do so, then we might as well forget about them until they turn up again. This is a hard doctrine—for, as we shall see, ancient testimony can be very persuasive indeed (and, in any case, if the laws of the known material universe *were* once broken in the past, then they remain broken forever; no amount of time can heal them again). Fortunately, however, all the major phenomena in question do occur quite frequently in our own time, here and now—so that we do not have to make the hard decision to refuse to pretend to study that which is not actually available for study. Given, though, that the same kind of events already reported in the past do occur in the present, we can then take a critical or at least a cautious look at the ancient reports, to see if there is anything to learn from them. The use of ancient material as supportive evidence is permissible, as long as we avoid offering it as sole proof.

Demons (of which incubi and succubi are one kind) are at least as old as mankind itself and throng in great numbers in the very earliest records. Generally they are said to live in lonely places—in deserts, graveyards, among ruins, and so on—and their power is claimed to be greatest during the hours of darkness. They are also likely to attack a human being who sleeps alone in a house. These, however, are the situations when we are most nervous. So perhaps demons are only as old as our nervous system, or perhaps they had some separate existence of their own before mankind came along. At any rate, reports of demons and devils are found among all peoples throughout the world,[1] and while at the edges such creatures sometimes blur with ghosts or nature spirits (and have even acquired, it seems, one or two characteristics from the pockets of Neanderthal men who have survived into historical times[2]), their "natural history" is rather consistent. All reports agree that demons prey upon mankind, to do him mischief. They are said to be "especially dangerous to women and children, and at the critical periods of life are alert to work them harm." (The "critical periods" are presumably puberty, menopause, childbirth, illness, and so on.) In physical appearance, while often humanoid, they frequently have characteristics of animals—horns, a coat of hair, pointed ears, wings, cloven feet, and so on. Sometimes they are fully animal.

Why should demons be especially dangerous to women and children? Nor again is it entirely clear why demons, which as a species are dedicated to preying on human beings, should inhabit desolate places. Without being dogmatic at this stage, we can say that the catalog so far is certainly as much one of human psychological states as it is of any actual creature.

However, the more detailed items we now go on to consider are *not* in any obvious sense attributes of the human nervous system or its psychology, at least not as these are currently conceptualized. The tradition of the incubus is principally found in Europe and the Middle East. Parallels are found also in Chinese, American, Indian, African, and other traditions, as we shall see, although the *overt* (as opposed to implied) sexuality of the European and Arab demon, compared with his counterpart in other cultures, is somewhat special.

Probably the best point of departure from which to survey our Western tradition is the nightmare (although this is also found as Yen Mei, the "nightmare demon" of China, the Anhanga, or incubus–nightmare, of the Amazon basin, and so on[3]). The second part of this term is the Old Germanic *mare,* meaning variously a goblin, specter, or hag. This creature was said to produce evil dreams (nightmares) by sitting on the chest of the sleeper. These dreams might be carnal in nature, or they might simply involve a sense of suffocation or oppression. There is in fact a continuum here, even though the two states at first sight appear very different (Sandy, in chapter 1, for instance, experienced both phenomena on the same occasion), ranging from light, mild, voluptuous sensations and caresses, to pressure, then to extreme and painful pressure. Folklore, at least, claims that such pressure can actually be sufficient to kill. So, for instance, the French, and adoptive English, word *cauchemar* (nightmare) means literally "the creature which tramples," from Old French *chaucher,* to "trample," in turn derived from the Latin word for heel *(calx).* Ernest Klein (*A Comprehensive Etymological Dictionary of the English Language,* Elsevier, 1966) gives the meaning of present-day *cauchemar* and the English suffix *mare* simply as incubus. Klein further notes that the general Germanic term *mare* is the same as the first syllable of Old Irish *Mor-rigain,* the name of the demoness of corpses, literally "queen of the nightmare."

The farther back we go in historical time the rapidly less figurative and rapidly more literal the nightmare becomes. (Even the scientific term for nightmare, *ephialtes* means in Greek "to leap upon.") It is the night*rider,* the *creature* that rides the man or woman to love or death. Our (self-protective?) use of the word nightmare simply to mean a bad dream is a recent one. Neither does present-day usage acknowledge the clearly carnal connotations of the nightmare (and, for that matter, of all dreams) that are seen in older texts—but that, however, Sigmund Freud has independently re-emphasized in modern times.[4] It should perhaps be stressed that normal human males have an erection of the penis, and females an erection of the clitoris, during more than 90 percent of the time spent in dreaming.[5]

Our central interest here, however, is in the fact that in earlier times the terms for nightmare and incubus are one and the same. The nightmare is the incubus or succubus.

Among the many accounts and depositions concerning incubi and succubi, perhaps the most startling is that in medieval times these demons were recognized not just in ecclesiastical law, which we might expect, but also in civil law and were often cited in court proceedings.[6] They were not considered to be hypothetical creatures; they were thought of as real.

Montague Summers perhaps best sums up the doubts that the modern mind has in allowing succubi and incubi some kind of objective reality—that is, admitting that something is involved other than hysterical hallucination or the agency of a real human being pretending to be an incubus:

It is obvious that there is no question here [as the witches claimed] of animal familiars, but rather of evil intelligences who were, it is believed, able to assume a body of flesh. The whole question is, perhaps, one of the most dark and difficult connected with witchcraft and magic. . . . In the first place, we may freely allow that many of these lubricities are to be ascribed to hysteria and hallucinations, to nightmare and the imaginings of disease, but when all deductions have been made—when we admit that in many cases the incubus or succubus can but have been a human being, some aspect of the Grand Master of the district—none the less enough remains from the records of the trials to convince an unprejudiced mind that there was a considerable substratum of fact in the confessions of the accused.[7]

This is heavy stuff, of course, but a good many respected writers of the past agree with Summers. Pope Innocent VIII in his Papal Bull of 1484 wrote: "It has indeed come to our knowledge and deeply grieved are we to hear it, that many persons of both sexes . . . have abused themselves with evil spirits, both incubi and succubi." And St. Augustus in his *City of God* (Book xv, Chapter 23) notes:

It is widely credited, and such belief is confirmed by the direct or indirect testimony of thoroughly trustworthy people, that Sylvans and Fauns, commonly called Incubi, have frequently molested women, sought and obtained from them coition . . . the fact is testified by so many and such weighty authorities, that it were impudent to doubt it.

What Summers himself is really asking in his various books is whether we are prepared to maintain that throughout the admittedly confused and uninformed Middle Ages and earlier there were not at least a few thoughtful, intelligent, dispassionate men who loved the truth, who could also sidestep the general hysteria and the obvious lies and conclude that *something* inexplicable was really going on. As we know, it was (is). The question is: precisely what?

A glance at some still earlier testimony.

The Babylonians had a panoply of demons. Among these were Lilû, who cohabited with women in their sleep, and his female counterpart Lilîtu, who did the same with men. These names are derived from Sumerian *lil*, meaning wind or wind demon. Rushing noises and the sensation of winds were already briefly noted in connection with some of the phenomena described in chapter 1, and are common to many forms of mystical and psychic experience (for example, the New Testament, Acts of the Apostles 2:2, when the disciples were filled with the Holy Ghost). Lilîtu, the demoness of the wind who seduced men by night, becomes the Jewish Lilith, the hairy night demon, "the most baneful and frequently mentioned of evil spirits throughout the history of Judaism to the present day."[8]

The following is an extract from one of the earliest surviving Babylonian texts concerning demons:

> He . . . whom in his bed the wicked Alû covered
> Whom the wicked ghost by night overwhelmed
> Whom the great Gallû assaulted . . .
> Whom Lamashtu possessed with a seizing hand,
> Whom Labasu overwhelmed
> Whom the Seizer fastened upon
> Whom the Maid of Lilû chose,
> The man, whom the Maid of Lilû pressed to her bosom[9]

These are the general attributes of demons. Words like "seizing," "snatching," "covering," "pressing," "holding," and "binding" occur again and again (*Gallû* from which we have our word "ghoul," means "to seize suddenly"). These characteristics are too widespread and persistent to be anything but a statement of accepted fact and, as we have seen in chapter 1, are just that.

We need but mention finally that the familiar of the medieval witch, and that omnipresent character in all the world's folklore, the vampire (who, likewise, "seizes at night"), are also aspects of the incubus–nightmare. The Chinese accounts of vampires and werewolves have remarkable parallels with the European versions of these stories—including the fear of garlic on the part of the former.[10] Here is an extremely ancient, universal, and consistent substratum.[11]

To quote Ewen C. L'Estrange[12] and Montague Summers,[13] briefly and respectively, on the subject of the vampire-familiar-incubus connection: "Witches that have no paps nor dugs have sharp bones for the Devil to prick them and raise blood . . . the Devil by sucking blood makes a pap or dug in a short time" and "each witch is assigned a demon . . . this familiar can assume either a male or female shape; sometimes he appears as a full-grown man, sometimes as a satyr . . . and if it is a woman who has been received as a witch he generally assumes the form of a rank buck-goat."

It is tempting to linger with such items, but we need to move on both to the present day and to more solid matters, which cannot be said to be "merely in the mind"—where at least the side effects of the manifestations not only affect the material, objective universe but are visible to others.

Specifically, we begin to touch now upon the poltergeist. A poltergeist is usually defined as an entity which makes noises, causes objects to move paranormally, and occasionally starts fires. The incubus–poltergeist connection is largely missed or played down by modern investigators and theorists (such as W. G. Roll and A. R. G. Owen—see chapter 3), but connection there certainly is, as the modern case history reported later in this chapter clearly shows. It is also very clear in older accounts, such as those of Coleti, Menghi, Sinistrari, and others. The term poltergeist itself is a modern coinage, dating only from the last century. There are numerous much older expressions, however—*folletti* (Italian), *follets* (French), *duendes* (Spanish), lutins (English), and most interestingly the Arabic jinn (plural of jinnee or genie). The Arabian genie, equally, is an incubus. Abu Sina (Avicenna), writing in the eleventh century, was the first Muslim theologian of any importance to insist that jinn are *not* creatures of fairytale, but are fact: "When annoyed they will pelt the folk in the house with missiles and utensils."[14]

Some specific accounts now follow. All translations are from Summers.[15]

Folletti make their presence first known in a house by various silly pranks and idle japeries. Trinkets and knicknacks belonging to the house and more especially to the person whose attention the lutin wishes to attract vanish from the place where they had been laid down, only to reappear shortly afterwards in another spot. These tricksters next annoy people by hiding in dark corners and laughing suddenly, or calling aloud as one passes; they will even pluck the sheets off the bed from sleepers, or tweak one's nightcap. . . . *Very often they beset tender girls,* to whom they manifest themselves as handsome gallants, hot young amorosos, who pursue them with obscene suggestions, whispering in their ears the most indecent words at unguarded moments. [My italics]

Again "young and female" are points of emphasis, an observation that modern research confirms. According to Coleti:

Not long since a country wench, accompanied by her father, came to consult me. She complained that she was persecuted by an incubus who had appeared to her more than once, but curiously enough under the form of a most unlovely and evil-favoured old cullion. . . . He often used, at suppertime, to carry off the slice of bread which had been cut for her, leaving the victuals of others untouched. A thousand petty persecutions followed. . . .

In physical appearance, the incubus can take a wide variety of forms—a dwarf, a giant, an animal or part-animal, or whatever. It can be very handsome or hideously deformed. The form or appearance of the incubus can be (a) culturally determined—you see what your culture has primed you to see, (b) personally determined—the projection of your own (secret) wishes, or (c) personally determined again—but this time as the projection of your own personal *fears*. In Freudian terms, however, a fear is the negative aspect of a wish; a fear or horror is a wish denied, repressed, distorted. At some level, the psyche still needs and desires that which at another level it denies. Hence the denied puts in an unwelcome and unpleasant appearance as opposed to a welcome and pleasant one. (These matters are considered in detail in part 3.)

Girolamo Menghi reports an incident which he observed himself. In Bologna in 1579 a wealthy merchant was plagued by "noises and extraordinary disorders." At first he and others thought this to be the pranks of the children, but it became clear that this could not be the case. Menghi continues:

> The lutin *had fondly attached himself to one of the servingmaids, whom he seemed to follow withersoever she went.* He even espoused her cause, and after she had been scolded for some negligence by her mistress the lady was slapped and pinched by him, her headress torn, and cold water thrown upon her as she lay in bed. When the girl herself began to take measures to rid herself of him he got angry, and suddenly stripped her of her clothes. . . . [My italics]

Apart from the fact that the incident concerns another young girl, the case is interesting in that it emphatically attaches the phenomenon to one particular person. No matter where she goes, the events follow her. This observation is fully borne out by modern research; it is *people, not places,* that produce the manifestations. Menghi relates that similar incidents occurred in the same city in the following year. Here the incubus was centered upon a young girl of fifteen who had come to a family to be trained in domestic duties. "But the lutin raised such serious disturbances . . . moving the heaviest articles of furniture from place to place with incredible swiftness . . . that it was found impossible by the good man of the house to retain the girl in his service. She was accordingly sent away, and at her departure peace was restored."

A final case, from Sinistrari, is a particularly apposite bridge to De Felitta's *The Entity,* involving as its does physical harm to the subject of the incubus–poltergeist's attentions. In some attacks the physical violence was (and still is) done to women who in no conscious way sought or encouraged the attention of any devil. They were thoroughly devout and prayerful women who threw themselves fully on the mercy of the Church from the outset, begging for spiritual and divine help against that which attacked them. These circumstances were very powerful persuaders toward the belief in demons as independent, self-willed, evil entities.

> First he took away from her a silver cross filled with sacred relics . . . then her rings and other gold and silver ornaments. . . . Next he began to strike her cruelly, and after each beating, livid bruises and discolorations were to be seen on her face, arms and other parts of her body. . . .

There are indeed more things in heaven and earth . . . and one of them is the story of Carlotta Moran, which reached its appalling climax at the West Coast University of California in 1977, as narrated by Frank De Felitta.[16]

THE ENTITY

The story of Carlotta Moran begins suddenly with two attacks, totally out of the blue.

> (a) One moment Carlotta was brushing her hair. The next she was on the bed. . . . Some knock, like being hit by a charging fullback, plummeted her across the room and onto the bed. In a blank mind she realized that the pillows were suddenly around her head. Then they were smashed down over her face . . . she felt huge hands on her knees, her legs, the inside of her legs which were pried apart. . . . She felt herself being torn apart in repeated thrusts. It was the cruellest weapon, repulsive, agonizing. It was ramming its way home. Her whole body was sinking into the mattress, pressed down, pushing down by this ramming weight. . . . There was a scream. It was Carlotta's scream. The pillow was smashed back on her face. This time she could feel the imprint of a huge hand, its fingers pressing through into her eyes, over her nose and mouth.

> (b) She was struck on the left cheek. The blow spun her half around,

almost knocking her over, and she put out her arm to brace herself. Then her arm was pulled out from under her. Her face was forced into the blanket. A great pressure was on the back of her head, the nape of her neck, pushing her down from behind. . . . A powerful arm grabbed her around the waist and pulled her up, so that she was on all fours. Her nightgown was lifted up over her back and—from behind—she was violated. The intense thing—the giant dimension of it—the pain of it finding so quickly the entrance and thrusting so fast inside, ramming away like that's all she was, that place, and not a human being at all.[17]

Over the next three months these remarkable and terrifying events were eclipsed by others still more dramatic, and we briefly chart their course.

Frank De Felitta has chosen to give this case a fictional form although it was a real-life event that befell an actual woman in Los Angeles in the 1970s and was supported by psychiatric and other public testimony. One would have preferred a straight documentary format. As Eric Shorter notes, reviewing the subsequent film in the London *Daily Telegraph,* the fictional form betrays "a certain fondness for mere sensation which leaves us wishing for a more documentary approach," though what is presented to us nevertheless remains "an exciting and troubling mystery." Yet even if *The Entity* had been a totally fictional account, involving imagined events and characters, it would still be true—in the sense that all the events in it are duplicated in numerous other authenticated cases of the present day.

On the occasion of the very first attack Carlotta was fully awake, sitting up and brushing her hair. The attack came without any warning, and Carlotta was in no sense directly or indirectly involved with any aspect of the occult. The incident therefore supports the view of the ancients that demons not only attack the wicked or feeble-minded, but are "entirely and gratuitously hostile to all comers." On the second attack Carlotta had been asleep in bed, so on this occasion the entity behaved more like the traditional nightmare (nightrider)–incubus. The first two attacks took place by night. Subsequent events, however, also occurred in broad daylight.

A few nights later Carlotta awoke from a dozing sleep with a premonition that "something" was coming "from many miles away over a broken-up landscape." She ran to get her fifteen-year-old son Billy from the next room. What followed almost immediately was a severe poltergeist attack, breaking furniture, damaging walls, tearing curtains. Carlotta, Billy, and Carlotta's two little girls, Julie and Kim, fled to a friend's house.

The next attack, some days later, occurred in Carlotta's car, when she was driving, by herself, in broad daylight. Voices screamed sexual obscenities at her, and the car and its controls seemed to be taken over—or, at least, she found herself being manipulated physically to accelerate and crash the car. It did in fact crash, at speed, through the shop front of a bar.

At this point Carlotta began to consult a psychiatrist. He initially diagnosed her as a case of conversion hysteria (see chapters 13 and 14), and at first she also believed herself to be suffering from delusions. Later, when Carlotta began to believe her monstrous persecutor to be real, she was rediagnosed as schizophrenic (see chapter 15).

Poltergeist events continued sporadically—toasters floating in the air, ceilings cracking, noises, and so forth—visible and audible to both Carlotta and the three children. The rape attacks continued, with the sensations of weight and pressure of the traditional incubus ("it got *on* me, and I woke up"). Carlotta was also physically abused; the psychiatrist himself saw the bruisings and markings on her body, including tiny puncture marks and the actual bite marks of teeth. (Puncture marks and bites from poltergeist–incubi attacks are, in fact, not uncommon—a further link with the traditional vampire.) The incubus spoke to Carlotta continuously during the rapes, and she *saw* it for the first time. "I had the impression it was a dwarf."

The general situation worsened, despite Carlotta's psychotherapy. Kim and Billy were attacked and injured by the poltergeist force (but not sexually), and Billy was struck on the wrist by a candlestick manipulated by an unseen agency.

Another major attack on Carlotta was not so much a rape as love-making. But she saw the incubus clearly. He was six or seven feet tall, greenish in color, facially Chinese. He was extremely muscular, like an athlete, and the veins stood out in his neck. His penis was very large. (The figure Carlotta described resembled a typical Arabian genie. Although the fact is not fully brought out by either the psychiatrist or De Felitta, the creature was in fact a sort of giant penis—the swollen veins in the neck very much recalling the erect male organ. This interpretation is further borne out by subsequent remarks.)

Carlotta's own parents had been sexually repressed, deeply religious, neurotic, and unhappy. As a teenager going through puberty, Carlotta had, consciously, known nothing of the body's sexual functions. When her periods began she buried her soiled underclothes in the garden, not knowing what else to do and unable to approach her parents on such matters. This type of disturbed sexual-religious syndrome occurs in many of the cases of severe personality disturbance that are examined in later chapters. In particular, however, the sexual symbolism of Carlotta's vision, as well as its actual behavior, implicates sexuality as a major force, probably *the* major force, in paranormal physical phenomena. The vampire is a lover; specifically, a consciously rejected lover.

Carlotta now began missing her periods. She had become hysterically pregnant (see again chapter 13).

Next an extremely violent attack occurred when Carlotta was staying at the home of a married couple. The furniture and walls of the apartment were very badly damaged, and her two friends witnessed the closing stages of the attack. The incident is important not so much because it was, once again, independently witnessed, but because it emphatically underlines the concept of "people not places." The "haunted house" seems to be a complete misnomer: what we have is haunted people.

There are three more points that will be found to be important in many other contexts. A relatively minor one is that of enhanced dreams. "*He* tormented her with strange radiant dreams that flowed behind her vision like a distant cinema, too awful, too lovely to comprehend." A second is that when photographed in or near her paranormal state Carlotta showed a completely different appearance from her normal self. Usually she looked nervous and frightened, as if eaten up by the environment or by her own secret fears. At these other times she looked luminous, soft, glowing, and sensuous. Her face seemed to be behind a gauze veil, which softened the features and made her eyes large and dark. Even her body took on a different shape. We shall come across remarkable fundamental physical changes of this kind in many other contexts.

The third point concerns the observations of a witness. Carlotta's boyfriend was present on one occasion when she was raped by the entity. In a subsequent statement to the police he reported that he could see, as it were, invisible fingers twisting and squeezing Carlotta's breasts. "Something" was on top of her, pressing down on her and forcing her legs apart. (So sure was the boyfriend of the presence of a being that he tried to hit it with a chair, but only succeeded in hitting Carlotta.) In other cases there are reliable reports of invisible hands "seen" pulling at people. The skin and the body are pummeled and squeezed exactly as if by hands, but none are present.

At the mid-point in Carlotta's sad story two professional parapsychologists became involved. They were initially concerned with recording, rather than resolving, the phenomena. It was they who took the photographs of Carlotta. They themselves witnessed the paranormal movement of objects and their own hair involuntarily stood on end. They finally decided to build a facsimile of Carlotta's room at West Coast University, install Carlotta in it, and attempt to trap the entity with liquid helium (for they thought it possible that the entity had some kind of objective existence). There was indeed a devastating attack, in the course of which all the scientific equipment was smashed. During it a number of university personnel actually glimpsed the entity—the salvaged camera film, however, showed nothing. The experience of these observers may have been a collective hallucination: they well knew what the entity was supposed to look like—and in some sense were expecting to see it. The more significant outcome, all questions of verification aside, was that Carlotta became totally psychotic and is now permanently hospitalized. Her attacks, in milder form, continue to the present.

In attempting to understand the phenomena discussed in these first two chapters we must first go yet farther into the bizarre and currently inexplicable—involving such matters as poltergeist attacks, paranormal fire, and the alleged world of the living dead. In chapter 3, we start to examine the experimental background that is beginning to verify and authenticate some of the "wild" and "utterly absurd" claims concerning such paranormal visitations and the astonishing powers of the human personality that have been made persistently throughout history—and which, as we have seen, are still being made by entirely responsible individuals today.

We pass out of the so-called paranormal and the occult directly into the quite undeniably real, though still very strange world of the disturbed human personality—and emerge finally into the altogether sober worlds of neurological science and normal psychological testing and assessment. The whole is shown to be a seamless garment, an unbroken weave. At no point can the fearful critic say: "Ah, here is the gap between the impossible events you describe and the real world." It is all equally real. It is all equally true.

PART TWO ⊕

EXTENSIONS

3
P⊕LTERGEIST

Professor A. R. G. Owen was Fellow of Mathematics and Lecturer in Genetics at Cambridge University (he has since moved to Toronto) when, at the beginning of 1961, he traveled to Sauchie in Scotland to investigate the case of Virginia Campbell.[1]

Virginia was an eleven-year-old girl who, according to her doctor, was passing through a very rapid pubescence. She had been brought up in Ireland, but her family was in the process of moving to Scotland. For the moment, Virginia's mother was living and working in Dollar, several miles away from Sauchie, and her father was still in Ireland. Also left behind in Ireland were Virginia's dog, Toby, and her friend Anna. Virginia was living with her aunt and sharing a bed with her nine-year-old cousin, Margaret—instead of having her own bed as in Ireland. Virginia's situation was somewhat stressful, and her complaints in trance bear out this view.

The events described below were witnessed, at various times, by the Reverend T. W. Lund, MA, BD, Minister of Sauchie; Dr. W. H. Nisbet, MB, chB, a physician; Dr. William Logan, MB, chB, another physician; Dr. Sheila Logan, MB, chB, DPH, the wife of William Logan, herself a doctor; and Mrs. Margaret Stewart, Virginia's teacher in Sauchie— as well as by several members of the general public. Professor Owen remarks that the individuals named are not only witnesses of integrity but also trained observers. It should be added that while it may benefit a pop star or a novelist to be associated with the paranormal, such association can be very damaging professionally for a physician. We must applaud the courage of the three doctors concerned in testifying to what they witnessed.

Here, in summary, are the events that took place in Sauchie in November–December 1960, as reported in Professor Owen's book *Can We Explain the Poltergeist?*[2]

Tuesday, 22 November: A thunking noise, rather like a tennis ball bouncing, is heard from the girls' bedroom.

Wednesday, 23 November: Mr. and Mrs. Campbell observe the sideboard in the living room move 5 inches from the wall, then move back again. Virginia at this time was sitting in an armchair near the sideboard but not touching it.

That evening, when Virginia alone was in bed but not asleep, loud knocks were heard all over the house. Several neighbors came in during the evening, and they also heard the knocks. Around midnight the Reverend Lund arrived. In Virginia's bedroom he found the knocking to be coming from the head of the bed, which vibrated when he held it. At this time Lund saw a large linen chest (measuring 27 × 17 × 14 inches) full of bed linen rock and raise itself slightly from the floor, then travel some 18 inches across the floor, before moving back again to its original position. Margaret, who had not been in the bed, now joined Virginia, whereupon there was a violent outburst of peremptory knocking.

Thursday, 24 November: Virginia was kept home from school. That evening Lund, watching in Virginia's bedroom, saw her pillow rotate from its original position through 60 degrees. Virginia's head was on the pillow, but Lund was unable to observe any way in which the child could have caused the movement. Dr. Nisbet also called at the house that same evening. He heard knockings and sawing noises. More importantly, he too saw a rippling or puckering motion pass across Virginia's pillow. He could find no way in which the child herself could produce this effect.

Friday, 25 November: Virginia had been kept home in the morning but attended school in the afternoon. The class was engaged in silent reading when the teacher, Mrs. Stewart, saw Virginia trying to hold down the lid of her desk with both hands. The lid nevertheless raised itself steeply on its hinges a number of times. Mrs. Stewart could see no way in which the girl could cause the movement herself. Then the astonished Mrs. Stewart saw an empty desk behind Virginia rise slowly about an inch from the floor. Then it settled down gently, a little out of its original position. When the teacher examined the empty desk there was no trace of strings, levers, or any other device.

That evening Dr. Nisbet stayed in Virginia's bedroom while she prepared to go to sleep. There were spells of knocking, even when Virginia lay on top of the bedclothes. From time to time the linen chest, which stood clear of other objects, moved distances of about a foot. (The chest weighed around half a hundredweight.) On one occasion the lid opened and shut itself several times. Once again pillow rotation was observed (through 90 degrees), and several times the rippling effect also occurred but this time across the bedclothes.

(Dr. Nisbet was eventually able to identify a cycle of events: quiescence, followed by movements of the pillow and bedclothes, then knockings, and finally the movement of the chest. At the point in the observed cycle when the chest was due to move, Dr. Nisbet took it to the other side of the room. Still the lid opened and shut several times.)

Saturday, 26 November: The puckering of the coverlet and the rotation of the pillow was observed and confirmed by Dr. William Logan.

Sunday, 27 November: Virginia, in bed, went into a trance. She was talking and calling out for her friend Anna and her dog, Toby. She was roused from the trance and taken downstairs. The Reverend Lund came at 11:30 P.M., and Virginia went back to bed. She fell asleep, and in her sleep again began calling out for Toby. She was given a teddy bear, which she flung from her, shouting, "That's not Toby!" She struck violently at the bedclothes with her hands.

These day-by-day events also continued at school. With Virginia standing next to, but not touching, Mrs. Stewart's table, a board pointer started to vibrate and move until it fell to the floor. Putting her hand on the table, Mrs. Stewart felt it vibrating. Then the table began to move, swinging in a circular motion away from Virginia and the teacher. (Virginia, standing with her hands behind her back, said: "Please, Miss, I'm not trying it.") On a subsequent occasion a bowl of flowers moved by itself across the table.

At one point Virginia was taken to stay in Dollar. Here the knockings and bangings resumed. In Dollar, Virginia also again went into a trance. On this occasion she spoke in a loud and unnatural voice (here, of course, she is beginning to behave like a medium), calling for Anna and Toby. In this state she began replying to questions put to her. The replies, however, showed "a lack of normal inhibition." Back once more in Sauchie, Drs. Logan and Nisbet together saw the linen chest move and the bedclothes ripple, to the accompaniment of various noises, and Virginia once again went into a trance.

All the events so far described were, as stated, witnessed by several individuals of standing. A series of further events was reported by the Campbells and the two children. An apple was seen to float out of a bowl, and a shaving brush to fly round the room. The two little girls were poked, pinched, and nipped by unseen forces. A house visitor was also pinched. Colored writing appeared on the girls' faces, only witnessed by themselves, but Mrs. Campbell saw Virginia's lips turn a very bright red three times in succession. On occasions Virginia's pajama trousers were pulled off or her nightdress rolled up. Footsteps were also heard.

The Sauchie case has been reported in considerable detail for several reasons. One, it is a very recent case that occurred in full public view, and in the presence of several witnesses of impeccable integrity. Even were this the only reliable case on record, it would suffice to demand a change in our current view both of the universe and of the nature of the human personality. Two, it contains the features of many earlier cases, some dating from the distant past—although there are plenty of modern ones too—which we can therefore take on trust.

Professor Owen himself has selected thirty-six cases from past and present that he considers equal to the Sauchie case. In these highly reliable cases he finds a ratio of two to one in favor of a female being the center and cause of the events, and a predominance of young over old people. The next case, however, concerns older people.

Two "honest and pious" spinsters were persecuted persistently from 1776 to 1785. Paranormal sounds were frequently heard—footsteps, snortings, breathings and snufflings, tickings and sharp reports. Various apparitions appeared—an old man's head, a little dog, and so on. Household objects and stones were thrown at the two women. Frances (the more persecuted of the two) was often pulled to the floor by invisible hands and her clothes cut. When the two went to bed, little scraping things seemed to be running over them. They were often nipped, and animals the size of a small dog leaped upon them.[3]

The nippings remind us both of the Sauchie case and of the legendary vampire. Nipping and biting to the extent that blood is drawn are described in several other cases, for example, in the Gemmecke case in Indianapolis in 1962. The "animals" leaping upon the spinsters also recall the actions of the incubus. Interestingly, Matthew Manning's father (Matthew Manning himself is discussed later) reported a similar event in 1967. "He had the feeling that a cat was moving on top of his bedclothes, and up and down his legs, trying to find a comfortable position in which to settle down. After it had apparently done so, he would feel a weight on his feet, although there was no cat." Mr. Manning had this experience "on more occasions than he cared for."[4]

A number of striking modern poltergeist cases are reported by Dr. W. G. Roll, the parapsychologist, in his book *The Poltergeist*.[5] For example:

At five minutes past midnight on Monday, 16 December 1968, I was walking behind twelve-year-old Roger Collihan as he entered the kitchen of his house. When he came to the sink, he turned toward me and at that moment the kitchen table, which was on his right, jumped into the air, rotated about forty-five degrees and came to rest on the backs of the chairs that stood around it, with all four legs off the floor. It happened in the twinkling of an eye.[6]

In 1967 another very striking case, with very extensive movement of objects, concerned Julio, a nineteen-year-old Cuban refugee shipping clerk. In this and other cases Dr. Roll was able to chart the direction and the strength of movement of objects at varying distances from the individual producing the phenomena. He considers that such a person is surrounded by a vortex of energy. Objects therefore tend to travel in a circular path—hence the frequently reported veering and swirling of objects.

Another celebrated case occurred in Rosenheim, Bavaria, at the end of 1967.[7] In the presence of a nineteen-year-old female employee in a law office, electric light bulbs exploded and light fittings swung violently. The telephone system registered hundreds of calls that had never been made. Later investigation showed that the numbers were somehow dialing themselves four or five times a minute. Pictures on walls rotated full circle, books fell from shelves, drawers opened by themselves. Finally a heavy storage shelf weighing almost four hundredweight moved from its position against the wall. No such events occurred when the girl in question was away from the premises.

Yet undoubtedly the most remarkable modern producer of poltergeist events is Matthew Manning. His case is remarkable for several reasons. First, an outbreak of poltergeist activity in his own house when he was eleven was followed by another outburst when he was sixteen and in a different house and also at the boarding school where Manning was resident. It is very unusual for poltergeist activity to be repeated (and then, as it has, to remain a feature of the subject's life thereafter). Manning is further remarkable in that he can also produce all other forms of psychic phenomena—automatic writing and painting, telepathy, psychic healing, and so on. Some of these items are discussed elsewhere in this book. Here is a brief sample of the multitude of poltergeist events Manning describes in his book *The Link*.[8]

On Thursday night we were subjected to the now usual poltergeist displays in the dormitory, and that night it chose metal coathangers to hurl around. The next morning nearly twenty of these were found on the floor. Many of them had been completely squashed so that they were little more than balls of heavy gauge wire. The activity now continued throughout the day, and seemed to occur within a certain radius of wherever I settled. During the daytime studies were interrupted in as many ways as seemed possible. Friday night it was broken glass again . . . flying about. Also during that night the wooden chairs beside the beds took to dancing and capered around the dormitory, colliding with anything that happened to be in the way.

Later in life, when a young man, and appearing before television cameras, Manning regularly caused the main camera to break down, the reserve camera also, fused lights on the location, and generally interfered with any electrical machinery that happened to be nearby. But still more importantly, as a young adult Matthew Manning has repeatedly produced poltergeist effects in test conditions set up by some of the world's leading scientists. At the conclusion of his own particular experiments Professor Josephson, Nobel Prizewinner for Physics, stated: "We are dealing here with a new kind of energy."[9]

Important and interesting though all the various displays of poltergeist activity are—and later in this chapter we shall show that many of these phenomena have been reproduced experimentally—we are still more interested in cases where individuals are attacked in ways that resemble the activities of the incubus, the succubus, and the vampire. The first of these cases is from the more distant past, but those that follow are of our own time.

The following account was written in 1761–62 by a Mr. Durbin, a friend of the Gibbs family, but first published in 1800. The two daughters of the Gibbs, Molly and Dobby, thirteen and eight years old respectively, were subjected to a series of astonishing attacks. Though differing on many points from the attacks on Carlotta Moran (chapter 2), they are equal in severity.

The children had been pulled out of bed several times as it were by the neck, in the sight of [their parents]. The children lay on their backs, and I saw very strong gentlemen hold each child under their arms as they lay on their back: they soon cried out that they were pulled by the legs. Major D. held Molly with all his might and put his knee against her bedstead, but he cried he could not hold her, the force was so great that he thought three hundredweight pulled against him . . . I saw the children . . . pulled to the bed's foot [about ten times], and both the Major and the other gentleman pulled after them, though they held them with all their strength, the children crying with pain. They felt hands pull them by their legs, and I saw black and blue marks on the small of their legs, as if hands had done it. I held Dobby myself, under the arms as she lay on her back, but I found my strength nothing to the force which pulled against me, and she was pulled to the bed's foot and then it stopped.[10]

Durbin himself also observed the poltergeist movement of objects, and traditional knockings were heard. On one occasion, as the knocking began on a table, Molly's chair was pulled back so that she almost fell to the ground. Dobby then shouted that "the hand" was on her sister's throat. "I saw the flesh at the side of her throat pushed in, whitish, as if done with fingers, though I saw none." A little later Molly was struck twice on the head with a sound that all heard.

Seven of us being there in the room, Molly said she was bit on the arm. . . . We saw their arms bitten about twenty times . . . their arms were put out of bed, and they lay on their backs. They could not do it themselves, as we were looking at them the whole time. We examined the bites and found on them the impression of eighteen or twenty teeth, with saliva . . . all over them in the shape of a mouth. We found it clammy like spittle and it smelt rank.[11]

The next day Durbin was again in attendance in the Gibbs household, along with three other witnesses.

. . . when Molly and Dobby were in bed: it again began beating and scratching. . . . Their backs and their shoulders were bit while they lay on them, which put it out of doubt that they did not do it themselves. I heard the slaps on Molly's back; I could hear the slaps of a hand very loud, but I could not see anything that did it. . . . Their hands being out of bed, I took a petticoat and covered over their hands and arms with it, and held it down close on them to defend them if possible; but they cried out that they were bitten more than before under my hand. I pulled off the petticoat, and we saw fresh bites with the spittle in several places, though we covered them so closely. Dobby was bitten most and with deeper impressions than Molly. The impression of the teeth on theirs arms formed an oval, which measured two inches in length.[12]

Another remarkable case, from the present century, displayed the traction elements of the Gibbs's case but involved no biting. The case is described by the Reverend Haraldur Nielsson, Professor of Theology at the University of Iceland. His account was written in 1907 but not published until 1923.[13] The events narrated were also witnessed and attested to by Mr. Kvoran, president and archivist of the Icelandic Psychical Research Society; Mr. Thorlaksson, a senior clerk in the Ministry of Industry and Commerce; and two members of the general public.

The producer of the events was a Mr. Indridi Indridasson, who, although only an adolescent, was a professional medium. At the time he was living in terror of an entity whom he identified with the soul of a recent suicide. This entity, Jon, had been described in séances as vindictive and wild.

One night, in response to the medium's appeal for help, a Mr. Oddgeirsson agreed to stay the night in Indridi's bedroom, with Mr. Kvoran sleeping next door.

During the night the medium shouts that he is being dragged out of bed and is very terror-stricken. He implores Mr Oddgeirsson to hold his hand. Mr Oddgeirsson takes his hand, pulling with all his might, but cannot hold him. The medium is lifted above that end of the bed against which his head had been lying and he is pulled

down on the floor, sustaining injuries to his back from the bedstead. . . . The medium is now dragged head foremost through the
door and along the floor in the outer room, in spite of his clutch-
ing with all his might at everything he could catch hold of, besides
Mr Kvoran and Mr Oddgeirsson pulling at his legs.[14]

Two days later Mr. Thorlaksson and Mr. Oddgeirsson spent the
night in Indridi's room. Objects in the room were thrown about and
smashed. Now both the visitors flung themselves upon the shouting
medium. By exerting all their strength they were just able to prevent him
being dragged from the bed.

While they were occupied in this "the table which was standing
between the beds was lifted and came down on Mr. Oddgeirsson's
back."

Later the same night the party decided to leave the house. But while
Indridasson was dressing he shouted that he was being lifted. Mr
Thorlaksson ran into the room, grabbed Indridasson and threw him
on the bed, holding him there. Then he felt that both of them were
being lifted. He called for Mr Oddgeirsson, who came running to
help. The latter had to avoid a chair which hurled itself at him en
route. Mr Oddgeirsson now threw his weight on Indridasson's knees,
Mr Thorlaksson being on the chest, and they managed to hold him.
While they did this the candlesticks flew in from another room, and
the bolster flew out of its place from under Indridasson's pillow.[15]

A Romanian girl, Eleonora Zugun, was taken from her home village
in 1912 to live with her grandparents in another village. Here various
poltergeist phenomena were observed—objects moving about, showers
of stones, and so on. The girl was taken to Vienna, where she was studied by a Professor Thirring. Later he was joined by Harry Price, the British psychic researcher. Price observed poltergeist movement of objects
in the girl's presence and the repeated appearance of bites and other
stigmata on the girl.

Subsequently Price brought the girl to London. A reporter from the *Morning Post* wrote: "Soon after I entered the room a mark was noticed rapidly growing on the girl's arm. As I watched it, it grew into a number of cruel-looking weals which might have been inflicted by a whip or a thin cane. . . . Within a few minutes the marks had disappeared."[16] Like testimony was made by Captain Neil Gow, Colonel W. W. Hardwick, Captain H. W. Seton-Carr, and Mr. E. Cleplan Palmer. Price himself remarked of the wounds that "they were first visible as red indentations —the white surround gradually becoming red at the same time as the indentations became white, rising in a thick ridge above the level of the flesh. The ridge became quite white in the course of a few minutes, and rapidly disappeared."[17]

The case of Mrs. Renate Beck, her mother Mrs. Lina Gemmecke, and Mrs. Beck's thirteen-year-old daughter is reported by William Roll.[18] The incident occurred in Indianapolis in 1962. Following the strange movement and breaking of objects around the house, Mrs. Beck felt a sting on her arm, and there discovered three puncture marks. Very soon after Mrs. Gemmecke screamed and clutched her arm. This now bore five or six puncture marks. Mrs. Gemmecke was similarly wounded on a total of fourteen occasions on various parts of her body, including beneath her clothes. The punctures numbered between one and eight. Mrs. Beck was attacked only once. One incident is testified to by a neighbor, Emil Noseda. "We heard Mrs. Gemmecke scream. She was sitting on the davenport, felt choked. Policeman saw skin pinched as if by fingers, pin marks came then."

Before leaving the question of attacks by poltergeists on human beings, one recent case, which she observed with a client during psychotherapy, is reported by a psychoanalyst, Mary Williams. It should be emphasized that this case was reported in the extremely respectable *Journal of Analytical Psychology*.[19]

Roger, the patient, was a handsome man of thirty-two. He had held a regular commission in the armed forces and had been twice decorated for bravery but had been invalided out after repeated hemorrhages from the mouth for which no explanation could be found. (Is there perhaps a link here with Sandy's mouth hemorrhage in chapter 1?) Prior to this incident Roger's history had been normal, except that from the age of six (!) he had been troubled by strong sexual urges. However, he had been ashamed of his "crude desires" which contrasted strongly with his vision of "ideal love." (Already here is a hint of the splitting-off of an unwanted aspect of personality which we shall see over and over again in chapters 13 to 15.) As an adult Roger had found women irresistible and was extremely promiscuous, though he never achieved full sexual satisfaction in his relationships, due, he felt, to his concern for the woman's needs.

One day he went to a séance with a girlfriend. Both he and others saw a "violet light." He felt sensations of fingers pulling his hair and hands brushing his cheek. In later sessions there were sensations of cold, thumps, and movements of objects. He began to produce automatic writing. Then, outside the circle, he would experience someone touching his hair and face, again the sensation of cold, and odd mental feelings.

Roger was now diagnosed schizophrenic and was treated by a Jungian psychiatrist. The psychotic symptoms began to recede, but as they did so the phenomena crystallized into traditional poltergeist activity. Raps accompanied Roger wherever he went, doors flew open, and he was constantly touched, as well as having his head seized and turned on a number of occasions.

Roger's fear of a further breakdown brought him to the Jungian psychoanalyst Mary Williams. Poltergeist raps, audible to both analyst and client, began in the very first session. They were very loud and random in occurrence. Then, while Roger was relating a dream, "the cupboard door in front of us opened slowly and silently."

In the third week, a number of raps came from the bookcase behind the patient. He reported that he felt the poltergeist turning his head, which jerked round several times. Mary Williams notes: "I could see his neck muscles straining, as if resisting a powerful force." She continues:

> Meanwhile the poltergeist was playing up every time he went to see his girlfriend, and tormented her in his absence. It tormented him too at night. It would get hold of him in bed, and hold him fast while it tickled his face and tugged his hair. And his mother was

hearing raps daily. . . . After a few weeks he reported that the last time the poltergeist had got hold of him it had seemed more gentle and had actually moved him into a more comfortable position. He did not resist this time and let it hold him.[20]

Clearly, the poltergeist was now behaving like a typical succubus, so we have here a very clear link between these two kinds of phenomenon. Mary Williams concludes:

It was only a few days later that it materialized again, and it was its last appearance. It came to him in bed and lay beside him. He felt it pressing up against his side, then it seemed to be merging with him, and he experienced it as loving and gave himself to it.[21]

With this event the psychotherapy was successfully completed. Roger now had a happy sex life and was for the first time experiencing full orgasm. No further poltergeist or succubus phenomena occurred.

In Toronto in 1972 a group of people interested in paranormal phenomena decided to invent a ghost and then see if they could raise a phantom of him.[22] Accordingly, they gave the would-be ghost a name, Philip, and invented a history for him. He was a seventeenth-century British aristocrat whose mistress, a gypsy girl, was burned at the stake for witchcraft, whereupon Philip committed suicide by jumping from the battlements of his castle. For over a year the group of eight (which included the wife of a Professor Owen) met and talked about Philip in order to feel they really knew him. Afterwards they sat in meditation in an attempt to raise him. Their efforts produced nothing. Then they read the two reports that are described below and changed their techniques accordingly. Within four weeks they produced rapping sounds from the table around which they were sitting with their hands placed upon it, and the table began sliding around the floor. They began asking the table questions about Philip, to which the table rapped correct answers in a simple code. Philip was talking to them. In due course Philip switched lights on and off at command and produced cool breezes.

In 1975 the group was invited to Kent State University in America for a series of tests by William Franklin, Professor of Physics. For two days raps and movements of the table were produced to order under test conditions, and the sessions were videotaped. One sequence shows Professor Franklin sitting on a floating table. Philip also again went through his paces on a Toronto television program.[23]

Several other groups have since successfully repeated the Philip experiment. (What more proof, one wonders, does the scientific community want?) The two British experiments that set the Toronto group on the right track were as follows.

In 1966 K. J. Batcheldor published his "Report on a Case of Table Levitation Associated Phenomena."[24] The writer and two others (all friends) met a total of two hundred times between April 1964 and December 1965. At these meetings, which lasted two hours with a half-hour break, the three sat, at first in complete darkness but later with a red light, with their hands on a table, concentrating on producing phenomena. Results were fairly rapid. In the eleventh session the table rose clear from the floor. The group was now also producing regular taps, scrapings, and soft thuds on chairs, on the floor, and on the walls. Batcheldor describes some of the later sittings.

> The simple table motions of sliding and tilting were capable of enormous variation: the table could glide slowly and silently as if on candle grease, or make a rapid and noisy excursion of six feet or more, causing the sitters to leave their seats and stumble after it . . . it could beat an enormous tattoo, quite disturbing to the neighbours when the table weighed 40 lb! Sometimes it would rotate about its centre, either slowly or so nearly instantaneously as to take the breath away. . . . As the sitting proceeded the movements of the table usually increased in power and extent. Under these circumstances it was often impossible to remain seated, and chairs were pushed back and we continued standing. Sometimes we had to go at a brisk pace from one end of the room to the other . . .[25]

Other phenomena that occurred in various sessions were breezes, intense cold, touchings, pulling back of the chairs, movements of objects in the room, and the "glueing" of the table to the floor so that it could not be moved. There were also two apports: a stone was thrown across the room and matches from the kitchen were sprinkled about.

The author of this paper was at that time a graduate psychologist. Today he is a principal clinical psychologist.

C. Brookes-Smith, D. W. Hunt, and two of their friends took matters a stage farther at the end of the 1960s, as reported in their paper "Some Experiments in Psychokinesis," published in 1970.[26] The four participants were, professionally, an electrical engineer, a photographer, a secretary, and a dental surgeon.

This group worked in full normal light and with a remote-controlled camera. With their hands resting on the table they carried on a normal cheerful conversation. Paranormal effects were obtained in the very first session.

Results were in fact rapidly produced: knocks and raps were heard, apparently from the table, at the first meeting. Tilting of the table occurred at the second meeting and, after a few sessions, the phenomena had developed into violent table movements over which no exact control seemed possible, and which indeed caused anxiety due to the possibility of injury.

These movements . . . included the rising of the table some five or six feet clear of the floor, its movement over the whole of the room whilst in the air, and a peculiar oscillating descent to the floor, sometimes quite gently, sometimes violently.[27]

Subsequently the group caused a lamp to switch itself on and off and produced breezes. They were also able to cause the table to "hop" in a given direction on command and to "dance" to played music.

Distressingly, it is reported that many of these successful experimental groups disband because they grow tired of producing the phenomena and cannot think of anything to do with the energy involved.

What an indictment of their imagination. They could, for example, have attempted to produce mutations in seeds or to hasten the growth in plants. They could have attempted to cure individuals with terminal disease—for there is good circumstantial evidence that the poltergeist power is the same energy as is used in psychic healing. At the very least the groups could have issued standing invitations to skeptical scientists and to the staff of scientific magazines, usually completely obtuse in respect of paranormal phenomena. Demonstrations to the general public would also have been of value, to encourage personal experimentation in this area. The more phenomena we have the better.

Poltergeist phenomena, then, exist. What we require is not further proof of them but an explanation of how they work and of their precise relationship to the human personality.

A further link between the poltergeist and the incubus–succubus is possibly provided by an experience of my own. The visits of my own succubus had for a time been interrupted by drastic changes in the house in which I live. The rooms below my flat, formerly occupied by peaceful elderly lecturers, were now taken over by students, with the result that the previous early morning silence was gone—the time when I entertained my paranormal visitor. However, one night I awakened from sleep to find a heavy pressure bearing down on my right leg. I was delighted at the presence of what I knew to be an incubus, and mentally I invited it to do something else. Suddenly the room seemed filled with a fierce breeze, in which the bedclothes appeared to flutter. I say "seemed" and "appeared to" because no one else was present to say whether my experience was merely subjective or genuinely objective. At any rate, this event, if objective, recalls the puckering and rippling bedclothes observed in more than one poltergeist case.

4

PARAN⊕RⓂAL
FIRE

The London *Daily Telegraph* of 6 August 1982 carried the news that "a woman walking down a street in Chicago burst into flames for no apparent reason and was burned to death yesterday." The Chicago police logged the event as a case of spontaneous human combustion, adding it to the "several hundred"[1] cases recorded in recent centuries.

In spontaneous human combustion "a person's body is reduced, sometimes within minutes, to a heap of cinders . . . unusual features are the speed and intensity of the process . . . and the way that it is selectively directed, for example, leaving the extremities of the body unharmed and sometimes not even damaging the clothes encasing the body."[2]

Unlike most of the phenomena discussed in this book, spontaneous human combustion is (albeit grudgingly) accepted by modern science. Science could hardly do otherwise than accept, in view of the police and medical photographic evidence presented at coroners' inquests (see, for instances of photographs, M. Harrison[3] and F. Hitching[4]). Dr. Gavin Thurston, a London coroner and editor of the *Medico-Legal Journal*, writes (in 1961) that "there are undisputed instances where the body was burned in its own substance, without external fuel, and in which there has been a remarkable absence of damage to surrounding inflammable objects."[5]

Science has no explanation at all to offer for the phenomenon of spontaneous human combustion. On the paranormal side, fortunately, there are cases where we can, at least cautiously, link the phenomenon with poltergeist activity in general and with poltergeist fires in particular. There are therefore some grounds for considering spontaneous combustion to be an "inner poltergeist"—an uncontrollable burst of emotional energy that cannot escape from the mind out into the environment and which in consequence destroys the human being producing it. Interestingly, we have no record whatsoever of spontaneous combustion generated by animals, just as we have no evidence of animal poltergeist activity. Here then are strong grounds for regarding these phenomena as by-products of the highly evolved, complex human mind.

Eyewitness accounts of spontaneous human combustion—we come to some detailed accounts in a moment—speak of "bluish flames" that can not only not be extinguished by water but are increased by it. There is, further, the remarkable fact that the amazingly intense heat generated tends not to ignite or damage adjacent objects, nor to spread into any general conflagration. In scientific terms, we might consider that what occurs in paranormal human combustion is that body water (H_2O), which makes up 70 percent of our physical structure, is electrolyzed into its constituent elements of hydrogen and oxygen, both highly flammable gases, which are somehow self-ignited. The water sometimes thrown over the victim is, it seems, drawn into the process, so adding fuel to instead of extinguishing the blaze. What exactly causes this possible electrolysis to commence remains a complete mystery. Nevertheless, electrolysis is an electromagnetic phenomenon, and so the reason for the fire's containment or localization might be the body's own electromagnetic field. Before examining one or two cases in detail, we should perhaps once more emphasize the quite extraordinarily intense heat that is generated in the process of paranormal combustion.

Mrs. Reeser was the widow of a doctor and the mother of a doctor. On the evening of 1 July 1951 she was sixty-seven years of age, in apparent good health, and living in Florida, a few hundred yards from her doctor son. Her son left her at 8:30 that evening, and her landlady Mrs. Carpenter looked in on her at 9 P.M. Mrs. Reeser was then seated in an easy chair, undressed ready for bed. At 5 A.M. Mrs. Carpenter was roused by the smell of burning. She found the doorknob of Mrs. Reeser's bedroom to be hot, frighteningly hot. When the door was subsequently opened, a blast of heated air rushed out. Mrs. Reeser was, apparently, not in the apartment, and the bed had not been slept in, but closer examination revealed the truth.

> Within a blackened circle about four feet in diameter were a number of coiled seat springs, and the remains of a human body. The remains consisted of a charred liver attached to a piece of backbone, a skull shrunk to the size of a baseball, a foot encased in a black satin slipper but burned down to just above the ankle, and a small pile of blackened ashes.[6]

Commenting on the case, Dr. W. M. Krogman, Professor of Physical Anthropology at the University of Pennsylvania, points out that only at the very high temperature of 3000° F do bones even begin to fuse or melt, let alone disappear altogether. He tells how he has observed a body burn for eight hours in a crematorium at over 2000° F, "yet at the end of that time there was scarcely a bone that was not present and completely recognizable as a human bone . . . they were not ashes and powder as in the case of Mrs. Reeser and numerous other deaths by spontaneous combustion." He goes on:

> Never have I seen a human skull shrunk by intense heat. The opposite has always been true. The skulls either have been abnormally swollen or have virtually exploded into many pieces. . . . I have experimented, using cadaver heads, and have never known an exception to this rule.[7]

Dr. Gavin Thurston wholly supports these views:

To burn a body at an execution, for example, as much as two cart-loads of wood are required: and attempts by criminals to dispose of a body by fire are notoriously unsuccessful . . . this is a well-recognized medico-legal fact.[8]

As Krogman hints, old-fashioned crematoria have to employ some-one whose job it is to grind remaining bones to powder after a crema-tion. Even following industrial fires, let alone house fires, the remains of victims, though terribly charred, are still recognizable as human beings.

In another typical case, nineteen-year-old Maybelle Andrews was dancing with her boyfriend Billy Clifford

. . . when flames suddenly burst from her back, chest and shoulders, igniting her hair. She died on the way to hospital. Her boyfriend, who was badly burnt trying to put her out, explained that "there were no open flames in the room—the flames seemed to come from the girl herself."[9]

In December 1966, in Pennsylvania, a local physician, Dr. John Bentley—or what was left of him—was found by a meter reader, who had his own key to the house. Leaning over a small blackened hole in the bathroom floor was the doctor's walking aid. "Alongside it was the sole, macabre remains of Dr. Bentley: the lower part of his right leg, browned by the heat, the shoe still intact." In the room below the hole was a small cone of fine ash, about 13 inches high.[10]

In London, in 1922, Mrs. Euphemia Johnson had returned from shop-ping on a fine summer's afternoon. She made herself a pot of tea and had consumed half a cup before she was overwhelmed. Her "calcinated bones" were all that was found lying within her unburned clothes. The varnish of the chair in which she had been sitting was slightly bubbled, and the linoleum beneath the remains was slightly charred: yet the heat generated in the consuming of the body must have been that of a furnace.[11]

The reality and strangeness of this particular phenomenon of spon-taneous human combustion are therefore undoubted. They must dispose us not to dismiss lightly the evidence for other kinds of paranormal fire. Before we move on, however, two points should be made. One is that, as all authorities agree, more women than men are the subjects of spontaneous combustion. To obtain a more precise estimate of the proportions involved, all the cases mentioned by Michael Harrison in his book *Fire From Heaven* were counted. We may assume that the cases were chosen not on any chauvinist or sexist basis, but on the grounds of their interest. Of a total of 35 cases cited, 12 involved males and 23 involved females. As it happens, this ratio of almost two to one favoring women is the same ratio as that found by A. R. G. Owen in respect of poltergeist activity.[12] A similar bias toward the female as originator of phenomena will be found in respect of all types of events bar one described in the present book.

The other point is the abrupt suddenness of the onset of spontaneous combustion; this is an aspect we shall have further occasion to return to.

The starting of paranormal fires during poltergeist activity is a subject already touched on in chapter 3. Probably the classic case that links this fire-raising activity with the phenomenon of spontaneous human combustion is that concerning the village of Binbrook in Lincolnshire, England.[13] The events in question took place at the turn of the year 1904–5 and were widely reported in the press of the day. They were also summarized by the Rev. A. C. Constance of Binbrook Rectory and a Colonel Taylor for the records of the Society for Psychical Research.

The events began at the rectory itself, and comprised objects hurling themselves about and, on three occasions, items near a "not very good, or big fire" bursting into flames. We must remember that in earlier times, in winter, most rooms in all houses had open coal or wood fires. While a skeptic might feel that open fires were the cause of alleged paranormal blazes within a house, such objection is altogether ruled out in the more modern cases and we may reasonably assume that at least some cases of paranormal fire in former times were not so caused. Indeed, in the present case, a householder in Binbrook, a school teacher, reported to the *Liverpool Echo* that she had found a blanket blazing in a room which had no fireplace. The focus of events next shifted to Binbrook Farmhouse. Objects fell from shelves and were moved around the house (much as in Matthew Manning's home). The farmer himself reported that he felt a strong sense of psychological pressure in the vicinity of the house.

Then the farmer discovered the servant girl, who was sweeping the kitchen, with the back of her dress on fire. She was at the other end of the room from the kitchen fire at the time, which was in any case protected by a fireguard (as open fires habitually were) so that no one could approach within two or three feet of it by accident. The farmer grabbed the girl and smothered the flames. Thus far there is nothing paranormal in the narrative.

However, the girl was in fact "terribly burned" and in "terrible pain." The hospital, approached by a local newspaper, confirmed that the girl was indeed extensively burned on the back and was in a critical condition. They agreed that the girl insisted she was not near the fire at the time of the occurrence.

Such severe burns are not readily consonant with the igniting of a dress which was in any case soon smothered. We need not feel over hesitant in taking the servant girl's experience as a case of *partial* self-combustion (for which there are several precedents in the literature). Moreover, not only have other female victims been observed to self-combust from the back—"some who, like the . . . New Hampshire doctor, see the flames beginning to sprout from between the shoulder blades of kneeling women"[14]—but the servant girl was the typically "lost" and emotionally damaged person (like Carlotta in chapter 2) that we find in many kinds of extreme parapsychological events (see also chapters 10 and 14): "Our servant girl, whom we had taken from the workhouse, and who had neither kin nor friend in the world that she knows of. . . ." She was no doubt the source of all the strange events described.

Sometimes the paranormal fire is outside the producing individual's own body. Since his twelfth birthday a boy in Budapest, in 1921, had been producing paranormal fires all around him. Irate neighbors finally drove the boy and his mother from their home. It was said that when the boy slept flames flickered around him, singeing the pillow, but not harming him in any way.

A similar case was reported in the *New York Times* in 1929. Flames were observed to play over a negro girl, Lily White, when she walked in the street. When at home her clothes were said regularly to burst into flames, as did her bedclothes when she was in bed. She herself, however, was not harmed.[15] This self-protective aspect also appears in the following case.

In North Carolina in 1932 a Mrs. C. H. Williams's dress suddenly flared up. She had not been standing near any fire, closed or open, nor any source of flame. Her husband and daughter were able to tear off the dress before Mrs. Williams was burned—or perhaps she was in some way protecting herself from the effects of the flames. Subsequently various other articles in the home burst into flames—a pair of trousers belonging to Mr. Williams and hanging in a closed wardrobe, a bed, curtains in an unoccupied room, and so on. On a number of occasions the flames broke out in full view of witnesses.[16]

Jennie Bramwell, in 1891, was a fourteen-year-old orphan adopted by a Mr. and Mrs. Dawson of Ontario. The child developed meningitis and while recovering from the illness would drift into trancelike states. In one of these she suddenly pointed to the ceiling and shouted: "Look at that!" The ceiling above the bed was on fire.[17]

This fire was followed by *several hundred* others, which broke out in full view of the rest of the Dawson family. Fifty fires occurred in the space of one day. While they were dealing with one outbreak at one end of the house, another would start up at the other. Even the cat caught fire while Mr. Dawson sat looking at it. The family insisted that the heat generated by the fires was much more intense than that of ordinary fires (an interesting parallel, perhaps, with the abnormal heat of spontaneous human combustion). A wood-paneled wall, for example, was instantly charred to a depth of half an inch, and the other side of the wall immediately became too hot to touch. At last Jennie was sent back to the orphanage, and the fires ceased forthwith.

Willie Brough, aged twelve, of California was said, in 1886, to start fires merely by looking. His family, convinced that he was possessed by the devil, callously threw him out of the home to fend for himself. He was taken in by a local farmer, who sent him to school. There, as the *San Francisco Bulletin* reported, five fires broke out on his first day: one in the center of the ceiling, one in the teacher's desk, one in her wardrobe, and two on the wall. The boy appeared terrified by the incidents. He was expelled from the school that same evening.[18]

These last two stories date from the end of the last century, yet it is hard to doubt them. Let us, however, return to the present day and to the question of general poltergeist activity associated with paranormal fire.

In the previous chapter much evidence of Matthew Manning's poltergeist-raising was presented. Here it is relevant to mention his ability to generate patches of very high temperature. In considering these events, which date from the 1970s, it is important to remember that they were witnessed and testified to by several of Manning's school fellows and the school matron.[19]

On one occasion Manning, another boy, and the matron witnessed, late at night, a patch of light glowing on an interior wall. This was warm to the touch, although the room itself was unusually cold. This light was self-generated—that is, none of the three could establish any normal source for it.

On another, more impressive, occasion Manning was wakened by a prefect and taken along to the junior dormitory, where they were having trouble. (By now, of course, the whole school was "used to," if that is the right expression, the numerous outbreaks of paranormal events that Matthew was continually producing.) Manning relates:

When I arrived the room was darkened and several people were in there, mostly prefects and boys who had woken up. The room was exceptionally cold and there on the wall was a pool of very bright light, which on touching was too hot for me to keep my hand on. . . . Another small junior dormitory adjoined the one we were in, and we went into it to see if anything was happening in there. Nothing could be seen immediately; the matron put her hand up against the area of wall that backed where the patch of light was manifesting in the other dormitory. She found it to be warm, as I did, and we found it becoming warmer, indicating that the heat was spreading through the wall. . . . In the other room the area had by now become so heated that I switched on the main light, fearing that if some action were not soon taken, the wall would begin to smoulder or burn.[20]

This incident, like the others, passed without actual fire being produced. The headmaster, however, understandably very worried by the threat of fire in a boarding school, determined not for the first time to ban Manning from the school, just as, long ago, Willie Brough had been banished for a similar offence. Ultimately, however, Manning's headmaster decided to let him stay.

How exactly might paranormal fire come about? The answer seems to lie in a continuum of activity, from "simple" poltergeist activity upwards. If an individual can generate enough projected emotional or psychic energy physically to move objects, then he or she can also cause objects—or, conceivably, atoms—to vibrate vigorously enough to cause them to heat up. (Indeed, heat is *nothing but* the atoms of a substance vibrating faster and faster.) The vibration eventually reaches a point where combustion spontaneously and suddenly occurs.

Paranormal fire and spontaneous human combustion may well be basically the same phenomenon. We have some evidence that those people who produce the one can sometimes produce the other. An example is related in Isaac Bashevis Singer's story "Henne Fire."[21] It may seem strange to invoke a fictional story in support of a factual argument, but Singer is faithfully chronicling the legends of his, the Jewish, people; and writers of Singer's stature are as addicted to the truth as any scientist. At any rate, in the story Henne both produces paranormal fire all around her, and finally, self-immolates. Singer's account of the blackened skeleton sitting in a chair itself only marginally singed, and everything else in the room untouched, precisely parallels the many modern factual descriptions we have of human self-immolation.

Spontaneous human combustion, then, may be the result of an individual at some point failing to externalize a critical buildup of psychic or libidinal energy (which might otherwise manifest itself as general poltergeist activity) leading to self-immolation. The analogy of an electrical charge failing to discharge itself, relatively harmlessly, in the immediate environment may not be too far from the truth.

In any event, external paranormal fire and general poltergeist activity are quite clearly linked; and, as we shall see poltergeist phenomena are themselves not isolated from general mediumistic and psychological events, such as automatic writing, clairvoyance and the sighting of ghosts.

5

AUT⊕MATIC
WRITING

Automatic writing, like mediumship as a whole, is frequently claimed to provide evidence for the existence of discarnate spirits, which are said to express themselves by this device through a human agent. Whether or not this is sometimes the case, there are certainly instances of the phenomenon where quite clearly no spirit is involved. Equally clearly, however, automatic writing is sometimes associated with poltergeist activity.

In the early part of this century automatic writing was also widely used as a psychotherapeutic tool in the investigation of mental illness. Like hypnosis, it then fell out of fashion in the shadow of the enormous interest in psychoanalysis, and possibly also because of its links with spiritualism. Neither of these was a very good reason for abandoning a genuine and remarkable phenomenon. Fortunately, there are increasing signs that automaticity is once more coming back into its own.[1]

Probably the most remarkable display of the possibilities inherent in automatic writing was demonstrated by Dr. Anita Mühl, a physician at the St. Elizabeth Hospital in Washington. She began employing the technique with hospitalized neurotics and psychotics.[2]

In automatic writing a person allows his or her hand to write at will, while consciously paying no attention to its movements, or even while consciously doing something quite different (such as reading a book). Two devices are often used to facilitate automatic writing in the first instance, the planchette and the ouija board. A planchette is a small platform of wood on ball bearings or rollers, with a pencil mounted on the front. The hand rests flat on the board. In the ouija board, there is no pencil, but the planchette (or an upturned glass may be used) on which the fingers rest moves round a spread of the letters of the alphabet, spelling out words. Dr. Mühl used a different device. She suspended the writing arm of the patient in a sling above the table, so that a pencil held in the hand just touched the writing pad.

Some of Mühl's patients wrote backwards, at enormous speed. Sometimes the whole sentence was written backwards, with all the individual letters also reversed. Sometimes only the individual words were written backwards, although the letters were not reversed, and the sense of the sentence read forwards in the normal way. Sometimes the first line of automatic text would be written forwards in the normal way from left to right then, without the pencil being lifted from the page, the next line would be written backwards from right to left, reversing all individual letters as mirror writing. An example of this particular phenomenon is in the form of a little poem.

Oboman who
eats little girls
on the gate post
lives up on the
gate post all in the dark
he jumps out at me

Much of the automatic material produced by Dr. Mühl's patients was (a) artistic in form—little poems, short stories, drawings, musical compositions and so on—and (b) often of a fairytale nature ("many of my subjects have given way without restraint to enchanting denizens of fairyland in the pages of automatic script"). It is probable that Mühl's patients were, latently, of above-average artistic ability; and this link between creativity and mental illness and mental disturbance is found in many contexts. (It looks rather, to express the point at its simplest, as if conscious + unconscious = creativity.)

Some of Mühl's patients wrote upside down (an interesting link here with Luiz Gasperetto, a medium who draws upside down, producing remarkable Old Masters allegedly under the influence of the dead artist concerned—see below); sometimes they wrote with both hands simultaneously, producing an entirely different narrative with each. One patient who wrote backwards displayed not only an amazing gift of recall, but wrote this recalled material with great speed. Mühl would read to this patient a number of paragraphs of a story that the patient had never heard before. Then, while the patient herself read aloud something entirely different (from a newspaper, say) her hand automatically wrote out what she had heard just once, spelling all words backwards, without errors! When subsequently asked to copy out a paragraph from sight as fast as possible using normal writing and spelling every word backwards, the patient's speed was eight times slower, and she made many mistakes. A brief example of this patient's writing illustrates the extreme bizarreness of the activity.

Won I ma a elzzup ot eht eye—ll'I yas I ma a elzzup. Rof eht hturt fo eht rettam si I ma a elzzup. Na eretsua nam emac ot eht esouh eh dais os.

Similar behavior was also elicited by F. W. H. Myers, using a normal subject.

An interesting experience was tried of writing with two planchettes, F. having placed one hand on each. I suggested this in order to elucidate the connection between left-handed writing and "mirror-writing," and fully expected that the two hands would write the same communications [although the second version would be written backwards]. To my astonishment, however, the communications, though written simultaneously, were different and proceeded

from different "spirits." . . . Whenever F. wrote with two planchettes, the left hand wrote mirror-writing. . . .[3]

It is clear, both from Myers's and Mühl's subjects, that if we *are*
talking about spirit possession, it would be necessary to argue that two
spirits could control a person simultaneously; however, in cases where
the automatic script merely(!) reproduces what has been heard, there
can hardly be any question of the activities of an alleged spirit.

Anita Mühl's own summary of her research work is as follows:

The surprising and unexpected variety of material produced by
subjects is simply amazing. Latent talents of which the [automatic]
writer is in complete ignorance of possessing may be demonstrated,
such as writing poetry or stories; composing music; illustrating and
designing; while aptitudes for arithmetic, history and geography
may be exhumed where these had remained peacefully interred
before. The writer may record lurid criminal stories well worked
out in detail, though lacking in his usual personality all traits of
criminality and cruelty. Another writer may reveal personalities
claiming to be delinquents and prostitutes which would quite hor-
rify the conscious personality. The writer may fluently express ideas
in a foreign language which he has forgotten he ever heard. The
subject may display a sudden facility for using the opposite hand or
for using both together and may even produce two personalities at
once, each making use of a different hand and each representing a
different sex. He may write mirrorwise with either or both hands
and he may write backwards correctly and speedily. . . .[4]

It is very interesting in attempting to relate this phenomenon to
current theories of brain function that *both* hands can produce mirror
writing and both do it at the same time. Writing or speaking a foreign
language that one cannot recall ever having heard is a topic specifically
considered in the next chapter. The uncovering of denied aspects of personality is another matter again—though both these last argue rather

firmly against the hypothesis of possession by discarnate spirits. Here, it seems, we are dredging up material from the unconscious. Mühl, as the psychiatrist in charge of these patients, used the material so obtained in psychotherapy—and in some cases was able to achieve the unification, or reunification, of these buried aspects of personality with the conscious personality that, for whatever reason, had rejected them. It must be emphasized however that this model of mind, in which unconscious material is considered to be once conscious material that has been split off from consciousness and disowned, though adequate as far as it goes, will in no way serve as a full explanation for the major phenomena discussed in this book.

However, Mühl shows that much of the automatic material produced by her patients contained items that were crucial to their mentally disturbed condition. When this material was explored with the patient, and understood by her, a lessening of mental disturbance followed. One woman who was having various sexual difficulties, and had attempted suicide, produced scripts containing "the most obscene and filthy language." These scripts were so appalling that they were never in fact shown to the patient. (It was, Mühl notes, most uncomfortable to see an adult woman "of such refinement and charming manner" expressing herself unconsciously in this obscene and depraved way.) It transpired that the patient had been taken frequently to a drinking saloon as a child around the age of five, though she had only the vaguest conscious recollection of this time, and of being put to sit on the knee of a particular man. Here was the source of the language. (Here, too, is evidence that we shall see again and again of detailed memories of language and ideas not consciously understood, but recorded as if on tape and film, from the earliest days of childhood. Nevertheless, a most important point is that this material is also reorganized by the patient's unconscious into new forms—and here the analogy with the tape recorder breaks down.) Mühl was able to explore with the patient "the many humiliations," some of them no doubt sexual, surrounding the saloon episodes.

Another patient, who did see her own scripts, also wrote what were to her obnoxious and unacceptable statements, which finished with the words "do not destroy this even if it is horrible—give it to the doctor and get the explanation for it, it will help." Here the unconscious mind, or hand, of the patient was indicating its own wish for integration with consciousness! In these cases we are certainly not a hundred miles from the phenomena of multiple personality (see chapter 14) and in fact one of Mühl's patients was suffering from this extreme condition.

The French psychologist Pierre Janet has undertaken a most interesting experiment.[5] He produced automatic writing as a post-hypnotic command. Under normal hypnosis, a subject, Lucie, was told that soon after coming out of hypnosis she would write a letter automatically, without noticing what she was doing. Later, while carrying on a casual conversation with Janet, she wrote:

> Madam, I shall not be able to come Sunday as I intended. I pray you will forgive me. It would give me great pleasure to come to you but I cannot accept for that day. Your friend, Lucie. P.S. Best regards to the children please.

When shown this letter subsequently, Lucie denied all knowledge of it and proposed that someone must have forged her handwriting. On a later experimental occasion Lucie similarly post-hypnotically and automatically multiplied 739 by 42 correctly whilst carrying on a conversation. (It is, of course, totally out of the question that she knew by heart the answer to this multiplication sum prior to the session—so the "creativity" of the automatic activity is clear; it is *not* mindless.)

A further experiment comes from the American psychologist William James.[6] The subject, Smith, who was not hypnotized, sat with his right hand on a planchette, with his face averted and buried in the crook of his left arm. After the writing had been in progress for ten minutes or so, James pricked the back of Smith's right hand some fifteen to twenty times. There was no response from Smith. Clearly, this hand was in a state of dissociation from normal consciousness. Then, as a control, James pricked Smith's left hand twice. Smith now asked why James had done that. James replied that he only wanted to find out if Smith had gone to sleep. Later in this session the right hand (on the planchette) wrote: "Don't you prick me any more." Smith was shown the statement at the end of the session. He remarked with a laugh that his right hand "was working those *two* pricks for all they're worth"—obviously he was referring to the two pricks on the left hand. Then, in a session a few days later, James asked Smith, this time with his left hand on the planchette, how many times he, Smith, had been pricked on the right hand in the previous session. The left hand wrote "nineteen times."

Ernest Hilgard, Professor of Psychology at Stanford, reports similar findings.[7] A blind student who was a good hypnotic subject (so much for those who believe that the eyes are the vehicle for hypnosis!) was hypnotized and made hypnotically deaf. Under this condition he could not hear anything except at the command of the hypnotist. When, as a test, two wooden blocks were loudly and unexpectedly clapped together by his head there was no reaction. Then the hypnotist said to him:

> As you know, there are parts of our nervous system that carry on activities that occur out of awareness, of which control of the circulation of the blood, or the digestive processes, are the most familiar. However, there may be intellectual processes also of which we are unaware, such as those that find expression in dreams. Although you are hypnotically deaf, perhaps there is some part of you that is hearing my voice and processing this information. If there is, I should like the index finger of your right hand to rise as a sign this is the case.

To the surprise of those watching—including the hypnotist!—the finger rose.

At this point the blind man asked the instructor to restore his hearing, because he had felt his finger rise in a way that was obviously purposeful. He guessed that something had been done or said to make this happen, and he wished to know what it was.

The hypnotist now restored the man's hearing and asked what he remembered. The blind subject said he remembered being told that he would become deaf at the count of three, and that his hearing would be restored when the instructor placed a hand on his shoulder. "Then everything went quiet for a while. It was a little boring just sitting here, so I busied myself with a statistical problem I had been working on. I was still doing that when I felt my finger lift. That's what I want you to explain to me."

Next the instructor thought he would try "automatic voice" (which is speaking without awareness, or at least without conscious volition). He rehypnotized the subject and told him that when he, the instructor, had his hand on the subject's arm, he would then be talking to the part of him that had lifted his finger. The other, conscious him would not know this. Placing his hand on the subject's arm, the instructor then asked the "finger" part what had happened earlier. Now the subject answered:

> After you counted [three] to make me deaf you made noises with some blocks behind my head. Members of the class asked questions. . . . Then one of them asked if I might not be really hearing, and you told me to raise my finger if I did. This part of me responded by raising my finger.

The hypnotist removed his hand (so that the "finger" part was switched off) and asked the subject what had happened in the past few minutes. He replied: "You said something about placing your hand on my arm, and some part of me would talk to you. Did I talk?"

There are many points here we need to note in passing for fuller discussion later in the book. The part of the mind that Hilgard was tapping is not really the unconscious mind as such in its true sense—it is, rather, an aspect of the conscious mind currently not in the field of consciousness itself. It was the "out-of-consciousness," but it was not the unconscious itself: perhaps we should use Morton Prince's term here, the co-conscious. (Hilgard himself calls this function the "hidden observer.") In some cases the co-conscious was not even producing new material; it was only reproducing what the instructor and others had said, although this had not passed directly through the consciousness of the hypnotized subject. The co-conscious, nevertheless, is not merely a recording agent. It is an active, instigating agent also—it can write letters and multiply large numbers together, for example. Yet these *are* logical, cognitive tasks that the conscious mind normally undertakes. James's subject, Smith, in one sense was only reporting on the number of pricks his other hand had received, but the hand did add an original protest of its own. His consciousness had not known about this matter, though his conscious *mind* had.

Obviously we are here beginning to make a distinction between "mind" and "consciousness." This distinction is an extremely important one, and plays a major part in ultimate explanations of the major phenomena we are examining.

Even some of Anita Mühl's patients were also sometimes only using other parts of their own conscious minds—those who reproduced material that had been read out to them, for instance. Of course *they* were writing this out backwards, although they had not heard it backwards. At first sight this reversal looks like a typical unconscious product—the night monster Lilith has her feet facing backwards, for example, as is sometimes the head of the Chinese vampire, and in the Black Mass the cross is hung upside down, the Lord's prayer said backwards, and so on. But it may be that we can consider non-emotive reversals as a function, a slightly unusual function, of the conscious mind. After all, if one runs a tape recorder backwards, that does not make either it or the strange sounds it produces an occult phenomenon. Perhaps the interaction of the two cerebral hemispheres might account for straightforward reversals (although both hands writing backwards at once can scarcely be called straightforward). As a rule, however, "explanations" based on the division of the two cerebral hemispheres are decidedly unhelpful, and often downright erroneous (see chapter 17). For example, how is it both hands write different narratives, when only one hemisphere has a language center? Some of Anita Mühl's patients were certainly tapping into unconscious contents (the unconscious mind itself). They were producing totally new, and even strange, organized material. The fairytale content of many of their stories is very much the kind of subject matter we usually associate with the unconscious mind, as is the sexuality of some of the other communications. A more searching question is not just exactly where was this material being prepared, but why had it *already been* prepared and held in storage (as can be proved in more ways than one) and for what purpose. The precise point of these questions will become clear later. First, there is no doubt that the stories in at least some cases *were* already completed prior to their being used. In one particular session, for example, what emerged automatically was clearly the *end* of a story. The beginning of the story emerged the next day, and dovetailed perfectly.

The material of "past lives" (chapter 7), of multiple personality (chapter 14), of automatic full-length novels (see chapter 9), of automatic painting and composing (see below), of the Christos experience (chapter 16), and of still other major phenomena likewise emerges fully formed, unrehearsed—and, what is more, *suddenly*—complete in all its intricate detail. Where had the material been stored before it was produced and what would have become of it if it had not been used? *It need not have been produced.* Some of those who volunteered for hypnotic regression did not believe that they were hypnotizable, much less entertain the idea that they would, on the spot, produce intricate scenarios of apparent previous existences, using strange voices, and so on. So, we repeat, where was this material prior to use, why is it produced in such sheer volume, and what is it doing when it is not used? (It is as if the brain has in it a country full of factories that no one has ever heard about, endlessly producing goods that have not been ordered and will never be delivered.) Only by finding an answer to these questions can we reasonably reject the discarnate spirit hypothesis in its full form.

Automatic writing is related to automatic speaking, automatic drawing/painting and automatic instrument playing/composing. Anita Mühl's patients exhibited all of these activities—the poems and stories were often illustrated with intricate pictures and designs, and many other designs were produced separately in their own right. These drawings were all the more remarkable in that some patients could not see the paper on which their hands were working, and yet heads got placed precisely on bodies, and whatever.

Major examples of automatic drawing, however, come from Luiz Gasperetto, a Brazilian medium, and Matthew Manning in Britain. Gasperetto, working very rapidly, sometimes with his eyes shut, sometimes using both hands simultaneously and sometimes drawing upside down, produces new "Picassos," "Rembrandts," "Modiglianis," and so on, that to the layman are entirely authentic. (A film of the medium at work has been shown on British and American television.) Art experts, however, say that they can distinguish between a Gasperetto and the real thing—which in no way detracts from Gasperetto's phenomenal abilities, although it somewhat diminishes his claim to be possessed by the actual spirits of the dead painters. Matthew Manning's exquisite Dürer and Beardsley drawings seem expert-proof, however. Unlike Gasperetto, Manning works slowly, with eyes open, and right way up. He does not claim that the spirits of the dead artists are working directly through him—in fact he finds this astonishing activity mindless and boring.[8]

Mühl's composing patients (like Manning) did not suggest that they were overshadowed by the spirits of departed composers, and their compositions were entirely personal to them. Rosemary Brown, in Britain, however, claims that the spirits of famous composers (Liszt, Beethoven, Mozart and so on) dictate music to her. This is given to her note by note, and she simply writes it down on blank music sheets. Her compositions are indeed clearly in the style of the composer allegedly giving the dictation, already a remarkable achievement in itself. Their quality, though falling short of the excellence achieved by Gasperetto and Manning, is "too good to dismiss lightly" and "by no means of negligible quality."[9]

Rosemary Brown displays some of the attributes of the medium: as a child she often saw angels and spirit figures and was sometimes able to find lost objects intuitively. Her direct connection with music was slight—she had little musical education but did learn to play the piano in a rather average way.

In middle life, as a widow with two children, she was visited again by one of her spirits who identified himself as Liszt. He said he wanted to dictate some new compositions to her. At this early stage he worked by controlling her hands—automatic playing. Her hands would play a few bars, and then she would stop and write the music down. Nowadays the single notes are "dictated" to her (a batch for the left hand, followed by a complementary batch for the right), and although this is in a sense a laborious process, Rosemary nevertheless works more quickly than composers themselves usually compose. "Her" work is now being increasingly performed, there are two LPs and two published volumes of manuscript music.

Automatic writing will occur in many other contexts. Here in conclusion its connections with poltergeist activity are emphasized.

The remarkable physical events surrounding Matthew Manning have already been described (chapter 3). What Manning discovered, however, was that the poltergeist activities around him ceased if and when he produced automatic writing and automatic drawing.[10]

The first instances of automatic writing in Manning's life were "poltergeist writing," a rare phenomenon. This took the form of "childlike" circular scribbles on walls throughout the house. Although they were done in the "lead" of lead pencils, as far as could be ascertained no actual pencils were being used at this stage. Then actual words appeared like "Matthew Beware." Meanwhile major poltergeist phenomena continued. At his mother's suggestion, Manning left a sheet of paper on the dining-room table, as an invitation for the writing to appear on it. On this and other subsequent sheets appeared scribbles, Manning's birth sign of Leo, and again the words "Matthew Beware."

Later, at boarding school, Manning involuntarily began producing "normal" automatic writing. While pausing to think in the course of writing an essay he found his hand taken over, and a flood of incomprehensible words produced. As a result of this spontaneous experience, Manning got together with some of his friends for an evening experiment, in which he allowed his hand to write at will. Bursts of fairly standard automatic product resulted: "I need help now. You cannot get me. Help. Please." Then, in answer to the question, who are you?: "Joseph West 1783. Get the dog. I need you to help soon. Fire."—and so on.

The interesting point is that after this automatic session no further poltergeist phenomena occurred in the school for the next thirty-six hours. Manning continued with automatic writing in the weeks that followed. The "messages" went on. "It was becoming obvious, though, that whenever I did automatic writing, the poltergeist phenomena would temporarily cease."

The remarkable content of some of the later automatic writing—which included many foreign language transmissions—is best considered under the topic of mediumship. But the notion that had begun growing in Manning's mind was that the "energy" which produced the writing and the poltergeist activities were one and the same.

> By December 1971 I had been doing automatic writing for nearly
> five months. Very little poltergeist activity had been witnessed since
> July; in fact, the only time such a phenomenon occurred was when
> I had done no writing or drawing for over a week, and then small
> objects would move about in a mischievous way.[11]

Summarizing the position, Manning notes: "Somehow I feel a build-up of kinetic energy. If I do no writing or drawing for two weeks or more, I become subject to poltergeist activity." Manning has frequently demonstrated his automatic abilities in front of television cameras, and the relationship between automatic writing/drawing and poltergeist effects is yet further underlined by the fact that Manning's appearances on television in this connection are frequently accompanied by major seizures and disruptions of the electronic equipment monitoring him.

Some further comment is necessary on Manning's automatic drawing. First, in respect of it he makes a casual remark that may prove to be quite crucial. Manning had been told by an automatic "spirit" communicant that he, the communicant, would get someone who could do a drawing for him. Two days later the said picture came through: *"As usual the drawing started in the middle of the paper and grew outwards in anticlockwise movements"* [my italics]. Anticlockwise is the natural movement for left-handers. Manning is right-handed.

The high quality of Manning's automatic drawings has already been remarked upon. What remains to be emphasized is their amazing range, volume and complexity. Dozens of different artists have drawn "through" Manning—Beardsley, Dürer, Rowlandson, Keble Martin, Bewick, Klee, Matisse, Picasso, Goya, and so on. (Some of these drawings are reproduced in *The Link*.[12])

During the winter of 1970 Manning had been researching the Webbe family, who had formerly owned Manning's family's house, for a school project. Now a Robert Webbe began communicating, first by using Manning's hand automatically—producing some fifty pages of foolscap. Then he began writing his own messages directly on pieces of paper. Finally, Webbe decided to "help" or "reward" Manning's research on his family by producing "half a thousand" names for him. Using Matthew's pencils, but only when the room was empty, the poltergeist Webbe produced, during a period of six days, 503 different signatures all over the walls and ceiling of Manning's room.

Quite the most remarkable example of poltergeist writing, Manning's phenomena, from the 1970s, validate the occasional mentions of this activity in earlier cases—usually involving writing on walls. Interestingly also, pencils were said to write by themselves on paper in the presence of the powerful nineteenth-century physical medium D. D. Home.[13] Witnesses to the phenomenon claimed to see a ghostly hand holding the pencil, but that particular aspect was, possibly, hallucinatory.

───── 6 ─────
PAST LIVES?

There are at least four kinds of "past-life" experience and possibly more. The kind that has received most publicity in recent times is that which takes place under hypnotic regression. In this method the individual is hypnotized, then led back by the hypnotist to his or her earliest childhood, even as far back as the womb—and then beyond. At this point, where normal memory ceases, the subject seems to cross some kind of blank divide, and then finds himself "remembering" lives that he has, allegedly, lived in the past.

Other types of past-life experience, which we consider later, are, first, spontaneous flash memories of apparently previous existences, which may be triggered by the sight of an old building or whatever, or simply just arise of themselves. Then there are the detailed memories produced, without prompting, by very young children, who announce that before they were born they were once someone else. Some of the material produced by these children is quite striking. Another, more deliberate, but very thrilling experience of a past life is obtained by adults using the Christos procedure (see chapter 16). This is perhaps a form of self-hypnosis. Fifth and sixth types are, possibly, the gradual recall in conscious adult life (but perhaps triggered initially by dreams) of very extensive memories of a past life or lives—this kind of experience has been widely described by Dr. Arthur

Guirdham in a series of books [1]—and the reporting of past lives through the use of automatic writing (as with the first of Guirdham's patients). These many forms of experiencing alleged past lives are not necessarily mutually exclusive: some people experience more than one kind. Perhaps the various, at first sight rather different, experiences are only subspecies or variants of each other. The personality type (and expectations) of the individual concerned may determine the precise form in which these particular creatures from inner space appear.

The evidence obtained under hypnotic regression in favor of genuine past lives is at first sight extremely impressive. From some points of view it remains extremely impressive even after close examination—that is to say, in itself it stands as conclusive proof of the amazing latent creative powers of the human mind, and equally of the living reality of the unconscious. The unconscious mind is shown to be no hypothetical construct or theory: it is a stark fact. Without exaggerating, we can say in respect of the regression experience that there are untraveled and infinite worlds of inner space that rival in every respect the limitless reaches of outer space. From all other points of view, however, there is very little hard evidence in the regression experience that any of us have actually lived any previous lives—although we cannot dogmatically and entirely rule out that possibility.

Under hypnotic regression events occur that are remarkable by any standards. The hypnotized subject quite suddenly and dramatically becomes *another person*—with a different voice, a different accent, a different facial expression, even, as far as voice goes, a different sex—who, more strikingly still, possesses a complete set of integrated memories about himself or herself relating to some past time, and to an apparent past existence.

Let us look first at the facial and bodily changes that occur in the regressed person. Ian Wilson writes:

. . . Mrs. Henry's apparent death is an example of the "facial blank," the total loss of expression and other signs of life that sometimes occurs in deep trance subjects when they switch from one apparent

past life to another. This is just one of a whole series of eerie and disturbing facial changes which may be observed during regressions. If
the subject is reliving a past life old age, the whole countenance may
take on a drawn and haggard expression. If he or she is reliving a past
life childhood normal adult facial crease lines may smoothe out. No
one who has observed these changes can fail to be astonished by the
sheer speed and subtlety with which they occur, as if at the press of a
button, with none of the adjustment that even an experienced actor
would normally require.[2]

There is an enormous amount that is of interest here. The sudden and
dramatic change of countenance and posture—well beyond anything even
the trained conscious mind can produce—is likewise observed in cases of
clinical multiple personality (discussed in detail in chapter 14). It is also
observed in mediumistic trance, when the medium is said to be possessed
by the spirits of those who have departed. Indeed, the behavior of the hypnotically regressed subject (which also closely resembles the behavior of
the severe neurotic suffering from fragmented personality) abruptly calls
into question the claim of the spiritualist medium to be possessed by discarnate spirits. The regressed subject is not possessed by a discarnate spirit
and yet is behaving just like a medium. Clearly, therefore, the onus is very
much on the spiritualist to say what (if anything) is different in the behavior shown by the regressed hypnotic subject compared with that of the
spirit-possessed medium. Obviously, something very real and important is
taking place in these various states, but do we—do we ever—in attempting to explain it need to invoke the idea of discarnate spirits?

Next comes the question, where on earth has the hypnotized subject
acquired his or her sometimes quite amazing knowledge of the past,
along with an apparently authentic accent and vocabulary? Such features do at first sight argue powerfully in favor of genuine memories of a
previous life. Yet is the knowledge of the past always accurate?

If a regressed subject, himself speaking in archaic English, is asked
about motorcars or television sets, he responds with the appropriate
bewilderment we would expect. Yet he has no trouble at all understand-

ing the modern syntax and vocabulary of his interrogator, even though this contains words and phrases that should baffle or at least mislead him; for language is continuously changing and evolving, not just in respect of idioms and colloquialisms, but in respect of the literal meanings of words. To take just one example, in Shakespeare's time "presently" meant "at once" or "now." To us today it means "later on." And then, what of the archaic language used by the regressed subject? Study of tape-recorded regressions by linguistic experts reveals that the regressed subject is using only a plausible-sounding *imitation* of an ancient dialect—the kind that modern historical novels and films will, incorrectly or at least inadequately, have suggested to him.[3]

In his book *More Lives than One?*[4] Jeffrey Iverson discusses a woman who regressed to a previous life as a Jewess called Rebecca in medieval York in England. She described among other things "the great copper gate" of the city, which she said she saw clearly. Subsequently, when conscious, she stated that she had no knowledge of the present-day city of York. Nevertheless, there is a street in York called Coppergate. However, this name originally means "the *street* (gat) of the *coopers* (or carpenters)." There never was a gate, let alone one made of copper.

Ian Wilson has written a first-class study of many matters of this kind in his book *Mind Out of Time?* For example, one subject claimed a memory of life in Thebes in Ancient Egypt in the reign of Ramses III and of using a sestertius coin. Ignoring the fact that this ancient Egyptian was speaking English, much else is wrong. Thebes was the Greek name for a city that the inhabitants themselves called "On;" and the pharaohs did not number themselves—this was a categorizing system originated by Victorian researchers. In particular, the sestertius coin did not appear for another thousand years after Ramses III.

Errors of this kind—often much less obvious than those just cited—can be shown by the hundred in regression accounts. Yet the real interest of the errors is not in discrediting the hypnotized person, but in showing us where the information used in the regression experience has really come from. The answer appears to be from books, plays, and films read or seen in childhood. (Here, surely, is a fact that must amaze us totally. It seems that nothing we have at any time seen or heard in the course of our lives is ever forgotten by the unconscious mind even if conscious recall retains no trace of it. Conclusive evidence for this claim emerges also in many other contexts throughout this book.)

Thus, Jan, a young female subject regressed by the hypnotist Joe Keeton, produced a most vivid and realistic account of herself as Joan Waterhouse, a young girl who went on trial for witchcraft in the sixteenth century and was condemned to death. This is a famous trial, of which we have detailed records. As her conscious self, Jan denied any particular knowledge of history (indeed, at school she had found history a difficult subject), let alone of the detailed published accounts of Joan Waterhouse's trial—and there is no reason at all to think that she was consciously lying.[5]

Jan's account, as Joan, was correct in every detail, save one. She gave the date of her trial as 1556, in the reign of Queen Elizabeth. In actual fact Mary was on the throne in 1556, and Elizabeth ascended to the throne in 1558. The real Joan Waterhouse's trial was, however, in 1566. When pressed on these two discrepancies, Jan as Joan spat back contemptuously: "You too say I lie."

Research revealed the following. The original Lambeth Palace chapbook, which carries the account of Joan's trial, was copied and republished in the late nineteenth century. The copier *mis*copied the date of the trial, writing 1556 instead of 1566. *This mistake was repeated in all subsequent popular accounts, stories, and plays* until recently, when the copier's error was discovered.

Thanks to this mistake, we can be absolutely sure that Jan's knowledge of the trial came from some account of it she had heard as a youngster (a story, a play, or a film)—and not from a previous life as Joan Waterhouse. Yet what an absolutely amazing situation we have here, in terms of the abilities of the human mind. A young child hears a play or reads a story, in all probability once only, yet her unconscious mind retains all the detailed factual information that the story narrates, without error.

The normal (not paranormal) origins of most if not all past life material are confirmed by another striking case involving a clergyman's daughter named Cynthia. The case dates from 1906, long before hypnotic regression became fashionable. Cynthia was hypnotized by a doctor in connection with medical research into hypnosis. In trance she began producing detailed past life material, apparently dating from the time of Richard II. The life Cynthia was apparently contacting was that of Blanche Poyning. Great historical detail and many names were produced concerning daily life at the royal court.[6]

This case came to the attention of the Society for Psychical Research, and was thoroughly investigated. The investigator, Lowes Dickinson, was impressed not only by the wealth of accurate detail, but by the fact that this was only available, in normal terms, in very obscure historical sources that Cynthia was unlikely to have read. The case seemed extremely evidential as paranormal knowledge. Then Dickinson hit upon the idea of talking to Blanche Poyning via the ouija board—a proposal to which Cynthia agreed. With Cynthia's hand on the board, Dickinson asked Blanche what was the source of her knowledge. She replied: *Countess Maud,* by Emily Holt.

Sure enough, just such a book existed, a very well-written and well-researched novel, which contained all the information Blanche had been using. Dickinson now took Cynthia back to the hypnotist. Under hypnosis Cynthia was asked when she had read the novel. She replied, at the age of twelve. But she said she had not actually read it! Her aunt had had the book, and Cynthia had browsed idly through it, and had painted one of the illustrations. She did not read it "because it was dull." Blanche Poyning was only a minor figure in the book. One important question, then, is why Cynthia's unconscious latched on to this minor character, Blanche. In other words (addressing the question particularly to western academic psychologists), who or what is the director of these regression scenarios—who makes the choice of cast, selects the camera angles, edits the story line?

On this point, and still under hypnosis, Cynthia claimed she had once met a real person called Blanche Poyning. This statement may or may not be true—it seems an odd coincidence. Perhaps Cynthia was closer than she knew to the condition of multiple personality, or perhaps this was simply a case of the unconscious weaving in some thread of its own devising, as sometimes happens in hypnotic recall.

Cynthia obtained her historical information and her basic story line from Emily Holt's *Countess Maud*. Did perhaps Jeffrey Iverson's subject, who thought she was a medieval Jewess in York, unconsciously obtain her character, Rebecca, from Walter Scott's novel *Ivanhoe?*

All of us have read, seen, and heard a colossal amount of information in our lives. (If a tape recording of the first twenty-five years of one's life were made, for example, it would take until the age of fifty to listen to it.) All of this information is, apparently, retained intact by the unconscious mind—even material that we have simply scanned in passing, or that is written or spoken in foreign languages! From this storehouse of material the unconscious mind endlessly spins stories and scenarios of its own, for what purpose and to what end we cannot guess, since in nearly all cases these never see the light of day. As Ian Wilson remarks, he has watched individuals known personally to him go under hypnosis for the first time, and reveal past lives as astonishing to themselves as to everyone else. Had these individuals not undergone hypnosis, where, we must ask, would the stories have been then?

Flash memories of past lives, as opposed to hypnotic regression, vary from vague feelings of "somehow I already know this place" to experiences where the person concerned momentarily, or even for minutes on end, finds himself quite literally back in another time. ("Throughout the centuries men and women from all walks of life have reported strange experiences when they seemed to see people, places and events through the eyes of another individual, and from times before they were born."[7]) These experiences often come upon the person while he or she is totally conscious and going about the normal affairs of life. They are of a quite astonishing, literal reality: one is *actually there*. I can speak of this aspect with great conviction, because I am fortunate enough to undergo such experiences myself, as described in an earlier book.

I was once visiting a museum in Jerusalem. In one corner of the museum an ancient arch and part of a roadway from some archaeo-logical dig had been reconstructed. Suddenly I was a young boy of about ten, standing under the arch and leaning against the pillar with one hand. My other hand was being clutched excitedly by my smaller sister. Past us along the road was galloping a troop of horse-men, seemingly Romans. I could feel quite clearly the clutch of my sister's hand. The noise of the hoofs and the clank of weapons filled my ears. Then I was back in the museum in Jerusalem. . . . Visiting an old castle and looking up at the outside walls I suddenly "knew" that I had been there before. Abruptly and momentarily I was in the thick of a siege. Arrows were pouring against the walls and shout-ing figures lined the battlements.[8]

Prior to the experience in Jerusalem I would certainly have doubted that Romans had ever ridden horseback there or anywhere else. Having since checked the point, I now know that they did. Perhaps I had once read a statement to that effect, or seen some film, but consciously I have no memory of it.

What is happening in these apparent returns to another time? It would seem that one's consciousness is momentarily displaced totally into the unconscious mind (that Aladdin's Cave of untold wonders) so that the unconscious itself becomes momentarily self-aware. (These are strange phrases, but as will be argued later, the unconscious may be a highly evolved mind without a consciousness. When we are able to invest it with consciousness—that consciousness whose job it is normally to service the conscious mind—then we achieve awareness of an alterna-tive reality, in fact of an alternative universe, some of whose names are fairyland, the Garden of Eden, the Dreamtime, Heaven, and Atlantis.)

A special case of the memory of past lives is shown by very young children. Two cases are reported by Nils Jacobson in his book *Life With-out Death?*[9]

(a) A spring day, before I had learned to talk properly, I found cracks in the drying earth in front of my parents' home. A memory surfaced that I had seen things like that before—and that the cracks had widened—and I knew that they were the first indications of an earthquake. I couldn't say "earthquake" so I screamed "the trembling, the trembling," but no one understood me.

(b) As a child I used eagerly to tell my brother, who was some years younger than I, what it was like "when I was big before in the world." I had a lot to tell, especially about America, among other things about when I was around when living people were thrown into a well (something which as far as I know I had never heard about). Later I read about the Aztecs and recognized my story exactly. The name Arras also existed for me even when I was very little; I kept repeating it to myself but didn't know what it meant. Later it disappeared, but the awareness that it was something special returned in the forties, when I heard the name for the first time.

These two cases might be nothing more than interesting curiosities but for the work of Dr. Ian Stevenson, Professor of Psychiatry at the University of Virginia Medical School. Stevenson has investigated and collected a substantial number of cases of reincarnational memories in children, mainly aged between two and six. The first fruits of his research were published under the title *Twenty Cases Suggestive of Reincarnation;*[10] Ian Wilson, who has extensively corresponded with Stevenson, summarizes as follows.

The child will perhaps begin to tell his parents, or anyone else who will listen, that he has come from a different home and different parents. Sometimes the claim will be set incongruously in the present tense: "I am the son of Shankar of Veheda," insisted one three-and-a-half-year-old Indian boy from Rasulpur. Such claims may be accompanied by a form of trance or delirium, often during the evening or early morning, when the child may relive, complete with a marked change of voice, episodes meaningless or foreign to the observing parents. Or the condition may occur by chance, perhaps when the child's family is travelling through an unfamiliar village. To the parents' astonishment the child may claim that he knows certain landmarks, and state that he has once lived there. He may even profess to recognise individuals and attempt to address them in an adult manner, as in the case of a two-year-old from Alaska who, being wheeled along in a pushchair, burst out "There's my Susie!" in recognition of a passer-by who was allegedly his stepsister in a past life.[11]

These children, it will be noted, are behaving very much like mediums.

What, at any rate, will probably impress the skeptic more strongly is that, according to Stevenson, some of these "reincarnated" children possess birthmarks and scars resembling the death wounds of those individuals they are said to be reincarnating. (So far, however, Stevenson has published no photographs of his cases.) The fact that these marks apparently exist, and sometimes bear some resemblance to wounds suffered by former individuals, is not a proposal we should necessarily choke over—although the explanation of such marks need not lie with reincarnation.

A famous case of scarring concerns the Pollock family in Britain. This dates from the 1950s, and has been the subject of close investigation and a television documentary. The preamble to the case is that John Pollock was deeply religious, a firm believer in reincarnation, and had repeatedly prayed to God to be given proof of reincarnation. Then the Pollocks' two daughters were killed in a particularly savage car accident, involving a driver under the influence of drugs. The children, Joanna and Jacqueline, were then aged eleven and six respectively. John, having recovered from the tragic loss of his two daughters, began to believe that they would be returned to him as a proof of reincarnation. He told his wife Florence of his firm conviction, which she did not believe. In 1958 Florence told John that she was pregnant. John immediately announced that she would have twin daughters, and that these would be his beloved Joanna and Jacqueline returned to him. Against considerable mathematical odds, Florence Pollock did indeed give birth to twin girls. They were named Gillian and Jennifer. Gillian was born first, by ten minutes, which made Jennifer the younger of the two. Jennifer had a thin, white line running down her forehead. Jacqueline, the younger of the two dead sisters, had had just such a white scar line, the legacy of a cycling accident when she was two years old. Jacqueline had also had a brown birthmark, resembling a thumb print, on her left hip. Amazingly, the baby Jennifer also had just such a birthmark. More amazingly still, since the new arrivals were identical monozygotic twins, the other baby, Gillian, did not.[12]

What are we to make of these strange circumstances, both the physical and the psychological, in this case and in the many others reported by Stevenson? A possible solution is to accept the correspondences described as real, but not to assign their explanation to reincarnation. (Wilson himself points to many internal weaknesses in the reincarnation hypothesis. For example, while there are many cases of poor children "remembering" a previous life of great wealth and status, there are no cases at all of rich children remembering a previous life of grinding poverty.)

One of the interesting features of the childhood "reincarnation memories" is that after the age of six or so the child ceases to have them, indeed loses all interest in having them, and typically as an adult has no memory of his previous memories at all!

Such a situation perhaps inclines us to wonder if some aspect of the nervous system has altered, an aspect that formerly produced the reincarnation memories. We do indeed have evidence of just such a change, from studies of child development. We know that around the age of five to six the nervous system of the child finishes maturing, leading to a sudden and dramatic acceleration in intellectual development at this time. Vocabulary levels, for example, that have been more or less static for the past few years, rapidly approach those of adults.

A possible view is that the mind of the very young child is open to telepathic and clairvoyant impressions in a way that the adult mind (with its "meddling intellect") seldom is. Of course, telepathy and clairvoyance will not suit western science as better explanations of the events we are considering than reincarnation. Yet there is ample evidence, both experimental and anecdotal, for the existence of telepathy and clair-voyance,[13] while there is very little for reincarnation. I have been sent many anecdotal reports by mothers of strong telepathic rapport between themselves and their pre-school children (a rapport that is usually sub-sequently lost). For example, a mother (as it happens, a social psychol-ogist) was sitting watching her small daughter and another little girl playing weddings with their dolls. The mother herself was wondering whether or not to go and see the film *Blood Wedding* that afternoon. To her astonishment she heard her daughter announce, "This isn't a church wedding, it's a blood wedding."[14]

As to the scars in the Pollock case, support is currently growing for the old wives' tale that the thoughts of the mother can affect the unborn child, and certainly that the fetus is aware and recording events.[15] We know, from their rapid eye movements, that fetuses spend much of their time in the womb dreaming. Are some of the contents of the dreams supplied by the mother? In a case like that of the Pollocks, where the wife was almost hypnotically exposed over a period of several years to the idea that her dead daughters would be reborn (even though she con-sciously resisted that notion), can it be that she unconsciously produced Jacqueline's scars on her unborn child Jennifer?

Before exclaiming "rubbish," those who would automatically reject such a possibility should consider not only the next few paragraphs, but also chapter 8, where, for instance, we have medical reports of adults who spontaneously and instantly produce on their bodies altogether real wounds suffered in childhood whenever they discuss those distant occasions.

Ann Dowling is a forty-seven-year-old housewife. She recalls, under hypnosis, the life of a nineteenth-century girl, Sarah Williams. This girl was, allegedly, badly beaten and finally murdered by an Irish navvy. Fol-lowing these hypnotic sessions Anne's body is, next morning, covered with real bruises. When Pauline McKay reproduces her past life as Kitty Jay, a Devon woman who hanged herself, the livid rope mark appears on her neck; and Edna Greenan, as Charlotte Marriott, produces a severe skin rash. Then, looking ahead to cases of multiple personality, as one of her personalities, Chris White, Chris Sizemore could wear nylon stockings without discomfort; but when she was Chris Costner, the same stockings would instantly produce an angry rash.[16]

The fetus is a part, a very sensitive part, of a woman's body. There seems no reason, *a priori*, to dismiss the idea that a mother could produce hysterical reactions of this kind upon an unborn child, just as she can upon herself. There does remain, however, the technical problem of the permanency of the child's scars.

Matthew Manning contacted the alleged spirit of Robert Webbe, the former occupant of the house in which Manning lived, by automatic writing. It was in fact once a common practice to contact the dead in this way. There are no immediately obvious objections to considering, at least as a strong possibility, the past lives produced in automatic writing to be an externalized or slightly more dissociated form of the same process that occurs under hypnotic regression. (Mrs. Smith, Arthur Guirdham's key past-lifer, also produced scraps of automatic writing in addition to her dreams and visions of her alleged past life.) The medium, who is "possessed" by the spirit of a deceased person, is perhaps a midway case: the possession is internal, in that the past-life visitor speaks with the vocal cords of the medium; yet the events are not fully identified with the consciousness of the medium—it is still a case of "his or her past life" not "my past life." Some hypnotically regressed individuals also remain conscious during the regression experience, just like some mediums. They then "watch" themselves as the past-life figure in a detached, passive way.

So, to repeat, there are no necessarily conclusive differences between past lives that are experienced direct and those that are the subject of communication in automatic writing.

A case of such automatic communication reported by Dr. Boris Sidis[17] is of interest not only because its story line so much resembles the exciting (seldom dull) tales produced under hypnotic regression, but because it is a good example of the enhanced and hitherto unsuspected mental powers shown by automatists.

Thus a Harrison Clarke, who began communicating through the automatic writing of a Mrs. Smead, showed "equal facility at inverted, mirror and normal writing." The inverted writing was from right to left and had to be read upside down. The mirror writing could only be read with the aid of that implement. In her normal state Mrs. Smead could produce neither of these kinds of writing. Harrison Clarke's long story was, in summary, this.

He was born in a town that is now a part of Chicago, and at two years of age was brought to Albany, NY, where he was cared for, until grown, by an aunt. He came first to New York City, and went thence to Baltimore, where he worked in a store until, becoming engaged to a lady and finding it necessary to learn a trade, if he was to marry, he returned to New York and entered the office of the *New York Herald* as a typesetter. The death of his lady-love in the meantime led to his enlistment in the army, and he was in the last regiment that left New York City for the [civil] war, and was in the battle of Shiloh, where, one morning after being out all night with his comrade, he was discovered by rebel guards and shot.[18]

It scarcely needs saying that all efforts to trace a real Harrison Clarke, even on the basis of this detailed history, were entirely without result.

Interestingly, Sidis includes Mrs. Smead's case in his book on multiple personality (originally published in 1904, but currently reprinted[19]) although few psychiatrists today would consider her to have been suffering from this condition—even if she did also receive communications from Mars, and believed her two dead babies to be alive on Jupiter! Such are not the symptoms of multiple personality. However, Sidis's judgment does nevertheless remind us how closely interrelated are all the mental phenomena we are considering.

In this chapter the similarities between hypnotic regression and mediumistic trance have been emphasized. There is, however, one very significant difference between the hypnotically regressed subject and the medium—and that is that the medium is also psychic.

7

HYPN⊕SIS

The general subject of hypnosis has already been raised, in the context of both past-life experiences and automatic writing. It will recur in many other connections also.

Like yoga and acupuncture, hypnosis was long dismissed by the Western scientific establishment as mere quackery and trickery. Its further association with other trance states, like mediumistic trance, was still another barrier to acceptance. Yet, as with yoga and acupuncture, hypnosis survived the sneers to become a major reproach to the adequacy of Western scientific accounts of man, and along with automatic writing and trance, hypnosis is becoming a significant research tool in the investigation of mind, psychology, and physiology.[1]

We must start by emphasizing the enormous potentials that are released by the hypnotic state, when induced in that 10 percent of the human population who are outstandingly good hypnotic subjects.

Probably the most daunting and famous case of hypnosis on record concerns a boy aged sixteen who suffered from a congenital, progressive, structural disease of the skin, present from birth. The condition, ichthyosiform erythrodermia complex, is resistant to all forms of treatment. In it, a thick, black, horny layer covers most or all of the body, and this layer itself is covered with further warty excrescences. The skin, if such we can call it, is as hard as a fingernail. Any bending or flexing of any part of the body causes painful cracks, which ooze bloodstained serum. The condition also gives rise to an objectionable smell that others find intolerable.

On 10 February 1951, in the Queen Elizabeth Hospital, the boy concerned was hypnotized and told that his left arm would clear of the disease. Five days later the horny layer softened, broke, and fell off, to reveal normal new skin beneath. In later hypnotic sessions the remainder of the body was successfully treated. The whole case was observed throughout by specialists and reported in full in the *British Medical Journal*.[2] One of the doctors involved emphasizes that *"icthyosiform erythrodermia* . . . is as much an anatomical mal-development as club foot."* It is remarkable, he adds, that it should respond to any form of treatment, but that it should respond to hypnotic suggestion "demands a revision of current concepts of the relation between mind and body."[3]

A physician who appeared in a British television documentary series on hypnosis narrated the following story. He was treating a boy who was suffering from the so-called "total allergy syndrome." These individuals have been described as being "allergic to the twentieth century." They have to be cared for in a sterilized, sealed environment and supplied with filtered air and special foods. The doctor was attempting to increase the boy's resistance by the use of hypnosis. At one point he began telling the boy that he (the boy) was having a picnic on a mountainside, but as the doctor described the imaginary scene, the youngster began to go into spasm. As far as his nervous system was concerned, the boy actually *was* outside in the environment with which he could not cope. The horrified physician realized that his patient was undergoing terminal spasm. Frantically the doctor now summoned up a helicopter, which swooped down and carried the boy up into the pure stratosphere above the earth. As the doctor quickly described these imaginary events, the boy's spasm subsided and he began breathing again.

This time the creatures summoned from inner space were able to mount a last-minute rescue.

Major internal surgery under hypnosis, without the use of anesthetic, is now almost a commonplace event. Such operations have more than once been filmed and shown on international television—and all this is taken as read as far as the present book is concerned. One other case, from the early part of this century, perhaps deserves a special mention.

Here the doctor concerned, a contemporary of Freud's, hypnotized a hospitalized hysteric suffering, as the doctor thought, from severe hysterical appendicitis (see chapter 13).

Under hypnosis, the patient described the sharp piece of chicken bone surrounded by pus and lodged in the appendix that she said was causing the appendicitis, and which she could clearly "see." The doctor suggested (still believing that the piece of bone was not real) that she manipulate her appendix internally, eject the piece of bone and the alleged poisonous matter, and pass the bone through her intestine to the top of the colon. Visible movement occurred in the patient's stomach, and eventually she reported that the bone was now where the doctor had asked for it to be. At this stage the doctor gave her a colonic water injection—and washed out the piece of bone that the patient had described.[4]

One of our more direct concerns here is with the imaginary events that the normal hypnotic subject sees around him at the suggestion of the hypnotist—and, specifically, with the imaginary people that he or she sees and interacts with.

The most interesting experiments involving imaginary persons are those where a real person in the room is duplicated at the suggestion of the hypnotist. One of the methods of achieving the effect is as follows. A selected person, X, has been sitting opposite the person about to be hypnotized. But while the hypnotist has been inducing hypnosis in the subject, X quietly leaves his seat and goes to sit behind the subject. Now the hypnotist reminds the subject that X is sitting in front of him, and instructs him to converse with X, which the subject does. Then the hypnotist asks the subject to turn round and identify the person behind him.

In this situation the truly hypnotized person is almost invariably startled, and will look back and forth between X and the chair where he has hallucinated the same individual. His behaviour resembles what is colloquially known as a "double-take." He will then identify both perceptions as X and may ask in a puzzled way why there are two of them.[5]

After a time, an intelligent subject—especially one who has some knowledge of hypnotism—may hit upon the idea that one of the two figures is a hallucination. He may try to test out this idea by asking searching questions of the two figures—but this tactic is of no use, since both answer questions adequately.

Before continuing the analysis of this situation, we must try to appreciate its implications. The normal, not the mad, human mind, under instruction from a hypnotist—that is, responding to purely verbal commands or requests—is able to fabricate an exact, true-life, free-moving duplicate of another person. Apart from being seen, this duplicate can be heard, touched and smelled by the subject. All the hypnotized person's senses are satisfied that this hallucinated person is really there, in the flesh. What a truly remarkable situation this is—and one which, of course, has all kinds of implications for the seeing of ghosts and spirits of the departed. Since the hallucinated person is after all not really there, why should we imagine that a ghost or a vision is? And is the famous incubus or succubus just such another hallucinated creature, a mere product of our overheated imagination? Well, matters turn out to be not quite this simple—there is the little matter of the paranormal movement of objects, for instance—but clearly there is much food for thought in hypnotism.

The hypnotized subject who sees two Mr. Xs cannot distinguish between them, even though he may have begun to suspect that one of them is a hallucination. Some bright individuals do finally hit upon a successful method of distinguishing between the two. Either by simply using their imagination, or by pretending to themselves that they have the power of thought transference, the smart subjects mentally ask the two Mr. Xs to raise one arm, or to leave the room, or whatever. The remarkable thing is that the hallucinated X does at this point raise his arm or leave the room or whatever. The real X of course does not hear the mental request.

Why is this situation remarkable? It is remarkable first because the hypnotized subject *cannot* cause the hallucination not to be there, in the normal sense. He cannot "vanish" the fake Mr. X—if he could do so, then he could not be hypnotized at all—but he *is* hypnotized. He is at the mercy of the hypnotist's suggestions—he sees reality as the hypnotist instructs him to. And yet he, the hypnotized subject, can himself suggest to the hallucinated figure that it raise an arm, or walk out of the door.

Here we have an important distinction between the hallucination produced by hypnosis on the one hand, and the incubus or ghost or equally the hallucinations produced by drugs on the other. The incubus, the ghost and the drug-induced vision do not do what we want them to, in any direct sense. They do what they want to do. The same holds for the visions of schizophrenia, psychosis, delirium tremens, and so on. The persecutory figures of mental illness have the sufferer at their mercy.

And yet, in the case of Ruth (chapter 10), most psychiatrists would undoubtedly have diagnosed Ruth as psychotic and hospitalized her accordingly. As it happens, Dr. Morton Schatzman did not. In time he was able to help Ruth face up to and relate to and persuade (although not always directly control) the figures that persecuted her—just as, indeed, patients with recurring nightmares can learn to relate to and to some extent exorcise the monsters that pursue them. This is a very difficult area, then, which does not permit of easy or glib generalizations.

Hypnosis is important because it begins to allow us some sort of controlled access to the otherwise often unfathomable and unpredictable.

There is the important matter, too, of minds within minds, or mental hierarchies. During extended experiments with hypnosis some of Ernest Hilgard's students (see chapter 5) became aware of the existence of what Hilgard calls "the hidden observer." As we already saw in that earlier chapter, there is a part, or parts, of the mind that hears, sees, stores, analyzes, understands, and acts upon information denied to the hypnotized person's consciousness, not only under hypnosis, but even after the hypnosis is lifted. Smith, in chapter 5, never knew consciously that his right hand had been pricked nineteen times with a pin, but both his hands could write that information automatically—and not just write the information, but comment on it! Some of the students became aware of this alternative activity of their minds that lay, and lies, outside normal consciousness. Some were quite happy about the situation, others were disturbed by it.

(a) I was surprised. The hidden part wasn't surprised because it was aware of its own existence, as well as the existence of the hypnotized part. The hypnotized part of normal consciousness was surprised because it's usually in the foreground . . . and now was shocked to be pushed into the background. It isn't used to that; it felt kind of betrayed.

(b) How can I be thinking and verbalizing something, yet doing precisely the opposite with my hand. . . part of my mind was observing both of these things going on, and was curious about them. I felt I had set up a conflict in observing this. . . . It's like a hierarchy.[6]

These students, perhaps, had begun to experience a one hundredth part of the condition known as multiple personality. In the second extract particularly is also a suggestion we have already met—that consciousness and mind are not at all the same commodity.

The remainder of this chapter is devoted to demonstrating how very little we actually know about hypnosis; and also to some evidence of a "conspiracy" dedicated to obscuring the differences between men and women in respect of hypnotizability. This conspiracy is actually part of a much wider movement in the west that seeks ultimately to deny the validity of all the major phenomena described in this book, and especially the existence of the paranormal, alternative universe of which they form part.

A single piece of original research by K. S. Bowers is itself sufficient to throw all our present conceptions of the nature of hypnosis, and the mind that produces it, into the melting pot.

Bowers[7] matched 36 men with 36 women for degree of hypnotizability, taking subjects at all levels of susceptibility, and tested them on measures of "creativity." It was found that for men creativity was slightly *negatively* related to hypnotic susceptibility, but for women there was quite a strong *positive* association.

Further experiment with most of the same subjects showed quite striking differences between the two sexes. Among all subjects whose susceptibility was relatively high, the relationship between creativity and hypnotizability was especially high for women and especially low for men.[8]

Anyone familiar with the general areas under discussion should on reading the above feel the previously firm ground shift beneath his feet. A *positive* correlation between hypnotizability and creativity for women is fine—but a *negative* correlation between hypnotizability and creativity for men runs totally against all our preconceptions. Surely creativity taps the unconscious mind, as does hypnosis? So how then can we have creative males showing resistance to unconscious influences? (Do we have to have two different models of the mind, one for males and one for females? It very much looks as if we do.) Reports of sex differences in respect of hypnotizability crop up sporadically throughout the literature. Ernest Hilgard, for example, reports a significant correlation between a favorable attitude to hypnosis and susceptibility to hypnosis in women, but not in men.[9] In other words, if you approve of hypnosis and are female, there is a strong chance that you will be a good hypnotic subject; but if you approve of hypnosis and are male, no such assumption can be made.

There are two lobbies in the literature on hypnosis. One (which includes hypnotists themselves[10]) believes that women are more readily hypnotizable than men, and another maintains that there are no differences between the sexes. What is actually going on here is well described by H. B. Gibson.

Weitzenhoffer[11] reviewed a number of studies on the sex difference in hypnotizability, later than Hull,[12] and noted regular slight superiority of females. We may wonder, therefore, why some authors state that there is *no difference* between the sexes. Here we come upon the point that may vex the lay reader and convince him of the old saying that there are lies, bloody lies and statistics. Some writers have the habit of saying that there is "no difference" when they have shown a difference that is "not significant.". . .

The fact is that if a certain tendency, however small, occurs again and again in the same direction in different studies, one can be pretty sure that there is a real tendency and in need of some explanation. . . .[13]

Gibson goes on to make a point that is also valid in respect of a lot of other data—for example, concerning the incidence of neurosis and psychosis in men and women respectively (discussed in chapter 13): with patience, one can find the data that confirms that neurosis is more common among females and psychosis more common among males; but the most recent study of sex differences available in this area was conducted in 1943.

Very little good work on sex differences in hypnotizability has been carried out, and because a somewhat mistaken feminist pressure in seats of learning has implied that it is somehow "wrong" to investigate sex differences, researchers do not always analyse their results with respect to sex as fully as they might.[14]

Gibson goes on to mention another important pressure on researchers —that of cost. It is much cheaper, for instance, for researchers to visit one college or school than to visit two. By lumping males and females together in one population, the researchers can more readily obtain enough subjects to make their findings statistically valid. If they begin subdividing by sex, and then, for example, by handedness they will necessarily have to visit more than one institution to achieve the required numbers. The pressures on researchers wrongfully to homogenize populations are strong. Some are conscious, others are unconscious.

Since they are also supported by the direction of other findings reported in this book, we can take André Weitzenhoffer's careful review of available research on hypnosis as revealing the true position. Weitzenhoffer finds that: women are more responsive to hypnosis than men; children and young people are more responsive to hypnosis than adults; neurotics are more responsive than normals; and normals in turn more responsive than psychotics and schizophrenics.[15]

On the question of sex differences, we have also the recent testimony of another influential researcher, Ruben Gur. He states emphatically: "One conclusion appears quite clearly: sex differences exist in correlates of hypnotizability, and these should be carefully scrutinized if we are ever to understand their implications for theories of hypnosis."[16] Gur has shown that the position with regard to susceptibility to hypnosis is far more complicated than has hitherto been suspected—as the title of one of his papers indicates: "Handedness, Sex and Eyedness as Moderating Variables in the Relation between Hypnotic Sensibility and Functional Brain Asymmetry."[17]

Gur felt that the inconclusiveness of studies attempting to connect hypnotizability with the believed importance of the differing functions of the two cerebral hemispheres was due to the conceptual naivety of experimenters. They had not only mainly ignored sex differences, but had taken no account of the handedness of their subjects, nor their eyedness.

The eyedness that Gur is referring to here is not that of which eye an individual prefers to use when looking through a telescope or a microscope, but another probably still more important piece of behavior. Experimental studies have shown that when asked to concentrate on a mental problem individuals habitually glance to the left or to the right while thinking. Contrary to earlier assumptions, it appears that it is not the type of question (i.e., whether emotional, mathematical, or whatever) that influences the direction of the gaze, but which cerebral hemisphere the individual is tending to employ at that particular moment.

Glancing to the right appears to be an indicator of the employment of the left so-called major hemisphere, while glancing to the left appears to indicate the employment of the right so-called minor hemisphere.

This terminology of major-left, minor-right hemisphere only applies to right-handers. Nevertheless, not even all the right-handers glance to the right most of the time! Some of the right-handed individuals Gur studied looked more often to the left. Similarly, some left-handers glanced more often to the right (which is equally unexpected); and yet others (both left and right-handers) glanced to the left and to the right in about equal proportions. In other words, handedness and eyedness did not necessarily agree; so which indicator should one use when attempting to judge which hemisphere is the major or preferred one?

This is only the beginning of the implications. For *all* females are "less well lateralized for hemispheric functions" than all males, and left-handed males also more closely resemble the female in this bilateral representation than they do right-handed males, particularly in respect of language function.

Given the situation just briefly described, the very least an experimenter can do is to control his or her study in respect of (a) handedness, (b) eyedness, and (c) sex. Yet even so, while sex itself may be a reasonably clear-cut variable, eyedness and handedness are not.

Gur himself reports two findings of interest. One was that individuals who were strongly left-handed (that is, used the left hand for all activities *and* glanced to the left when thinking more than 70 percent of the time) tended to be more readily hypnotizable than the pure right-handers; between the moderate left-handers and right-handers he found no differences.

Controlling for all variables (sex, handedness, and eyedness), Gur found *high negative* correlations between number of eye movements to the right and hypnotizability for right-handed males; *slight negative* correlation between number of eye movements to the right and hypnotizability for left-handed males; *slight positive* correlation between number of eye movements to the right and hypnotizability for right-handed females; and *high positive* correlation between number of eye movements to the right and hypnotizability for left-handed females.

This is all very baffling. Right-handed males who glance often to the right are hard to hypnotize (as a rule). But right-handed females who glance often to the right are indicating a slight positive tendency toward hypnotizability. But left-handed females who glance often to the right (which they should not be doing!) are very significantly hypnotizable.

Needless to say, the above findings are in respect of *group averages*. A right-handed, right-glancing male *individual* is not necessarily hard to hypnotize, and a left-handed, right-glancing female *individual* is not necessarily easy to hypnotize.

Gur's service has been to indicate the very great complexity of the relationship between nervous system characteristics and hypnotizability; to draw attention once again to the fact that males and females differ basically in respect of their representation of brain laterality (as do left-handed males also); and finally to raise again the whole question of handedness, with particular emphasis on left-handedness. This last issue is especially welcome—for, as we shall see in chapter 11, there is a very widespread censorship in modern western psychology on the entire question of the psychological and physiological characteristics of left-handers.

8

STIGMATA

An army officer of thirty-five was admitted to hospital for treatment for persistent sleepwalking, which he had displayed all his life. Some ten years earlier he had been hospitalized for observation of this same condition, on which occasion the doctors had tied his arms behind his back in the hope of preventing further somnambulism. Nevertheless, he had sleepwalked, but in the struggle to get his arms free he injured his wrists so badly that they were wealed and bleeding. Now, ten years later, he was administered the drug Evipan in the course of psychotherapy, but not on this occasion restrained in any way. The patient went into a dissociated state and began reciting fragments of poetry. Then he placed his arms behind his back and began struggling and gasping. Under the eyes of the doctor (R. L. Moody) the welts and bleeding of ten years earlier spontaneously reappeared. Photographs of the incident were taken, and appeared with a full report in *The Lancet*.[1]

Another patient, a woman of thirty-seven, had undergone a nervous breakdown. During psychotherapy she went into a state of mental dissociation, and in this trancelike condition was able to speak in detail of the dreadful beatings her father had given her as a child. As she described the prolonged and frequent scourgings, bleeding whip marks appeared on her legs, buttocks, shoulders and hands. These were witnessed, photographed and reported by physicians, and had moreover to be dressed and treated like normal wounds. Two further cases of this same phenomenon are also reported by Dr. Moody in the same paper.

These two cases show obvious parallels with the religious stigmata or "wounds of Christ" that deeply devout Christians and saints sometimes produce upon their bodies, which mimic the wounds allegedly suffered by Christ on the cross. The wounds of the religious stigmatic, however, unlike those of the psychiatric patients described, are alleged to arise from the overshadowing of the human personality by that of Christ himself; whereas "all" that the psychiatric patients have done is to reproduce from somewhere in their memory vaults—or rather, have perhaps caused to live again—the bleeding, suffering child or person they had once been.

We move a good step closer to the religious stigmatic in the case of a woman whose own hip began to bleed whenever she saw her handicapped son putting on his hip brace.[2] Here the source of the wound—or at any rate, the inspiration of it—is external to the sufferer, rather in the way that the suffering Christ is external to the religious stigmatic.

However, the argument for the wounds of the stigmatic (the spear wound in the side, the marks of the thorns on the head, the nail marks in feet and hands, and so on) having been produced by contact with the actual spirit of Christ collapses completely on examination. For example, the stigmatics regularly produced (and produce to this day) nail wounds in the palms of their hands as shown in the many paintings and carvings of the crucified Christ—whereas in fact the real historical Christ, like all crucified victims of those days, was nailed to the cross through the wrists. More telling still is the finding that the particular marks (size, shape, position) on some stigmatics are identical with those on the particular crucifix or painting before which the stigmatic habitually worships. Here we seem to identify the *exact* source of inspiration that the unconscious mind has employed.[3]

A twentieth-century stigmatic was the German Theresa Neumann, who died in 1962. She not only readily developed the traditional nail wounds and so on, but would weep tears of blood.[4] (She would also go into visionary trances and speak in different voices—phenomena with which we have already become familiar.) This wonder of weeping blood was, however, induced experimentally in another German girl, Elizabeth K., by the psychiatrist Alfred Lechler.[5]

Elizabeth (whom the psychiatrist employed in his own home as a domestic servant) suffered from the fragmented psychological condition known as multiple personality (see chapter 14). She was also prone to develop the physical symptoms of illnesses she saw or heard of around her—tuberculosis, hernia, and so forth. One day Elizabeth returned to the psychiatrist's home from a Good Friday lecture illustrated with lantern slides. She claimed to have severe pains in her hands and feet. Lechler decided on an experiment. He hypnotized Elizabeth, but instead of telling her that the pains would go away, he told her to concentrate on the idea of them getting worse and of real nails being forced into her extremities. The next morning Elizabeth was in considerable pain and had red, swollen, weeping marks in the palms (as usual!) of her hands and in her feet.

Lechler explained to her that he had caused the marks to appear in order to help him understand her psychological condition; he now asked for her permission to conduct further experiments, which she gave. He reminded her of Theresa Neumann's ability to weep tears of blood, and asked Elizabeth, as she went about her work, to take Theresa's troubles upon herself. A few hours later Elizabeth presented herself with blood welling from her eyes (a process that Lechler at once photographed). In later experiments, the mere suggestion in the evening of a crown of thorns produced puncture wounds in Elizabeth's forehead by morning. These could be made to bleed on Lechler's command.

The similarities between the phenomena produced by the religious stigmatics as well as by psychiatric patients, and the physical phenomena produced by some "past lifers" (chapter 6), and by other subjects in perfectly straightforward hypnotic trance (chapter 7), need no underlining. The parallels are clear—what we can describe as real wounds are, however, produced on the basis of suggestion only. We need not doubt that the same basic physiological–psychological mechanisms underlie all the cases in question. The apparent differences between them rest almost entirely on the claims made by the conscious personalities of those involved: past lifers believe they have brought their wounds with them from a previous existence, stigmatics believe they have contacted the spirit of Christ, and so on. But "all" that has really happened in each case is that each has brought forth a "wish creature" from inner space. *That* is the remarkable achievement, and the one with which we are concerned in this book.

One final firm link between stigmatism and past lives. Lechler asked Elizabeth to think herself back to the time of the Crucifixion. This she first did without any hypnosis, and produced a typical, vivid past-life experience of herself as one of the thieves crucified along with Christ. Later, under actual hypnosis, she "returned" as one of the children Christ knew. Again the narrative showed all the vividness, the clever acting and rich imagery we typically associate with the outstanding regression experience.

Elizabeth was, in addition, a diagnosed case of multiple personality. All in all then, we have in her a very firm bridge between many of the (at first sight) seemingly very different phenomena we are studying.

---9---

MEDIUMSHIP

Mediumship is from several points of view a very real phenomenon. The gifted medium, in particular, undergoes changes and produces physical events for which modern psychology has no explanation. Probably for this reason the subject is not mentioned in psychology textbooks.

In what we might call standard mediumship, the medium, who can be either male or female, lapses into a trance state and is then "taken over" by another personality, in fact a series of personalities, who are said to be the spirits of the dead using the physical body of the medium to communicate with us on earth. In passing, it must be stressed that although Spiritualism in Europe and America dates only from the second half of the nineteenth century, the phenomenon of such spirit possession is reported worldwide from the dawn of history.

In full trance dramatic changes occur in the facial expression, bodily posture and voice of the medium. The facial changes in particular go well beyond any power of acting. As myriad witnesses, myself included, testify, one really seems to be looking at the face of a different person. Even the bone structure seems to change (though no doubt it is only the flesh and muscle) so that one could swear one were looking at a Chinese man or a Native American or whatever. Nevertheless, such deep changes are also observed in hypnotic regression (chapter 6) and in cases of multiple personality (chapter 14). In these latter situations, importantly, there is no question of the presence of or the possession by discarnate spirits. On the sole basis of the admittedly dramatic facial and bodily changes alone, there is, therefore, no pressure for us to accept the Spiritualists' account of what is happening to the medium. I myself developed as a medium at one time, so that I can speak with some knowledge of what takes place internally during trance. When I surrender myself to the trance state, the first reaction is a slight feeling of light-headedness. Then I find myself taking sudden deep breaths that are not of my own initiating. My head may loll backwards, or perhaps slump forwards. It is then that another personality manifests itself. My voice begins speaking, perhaps a little hesitantly at first, yet I am not consciously speaking. My voice is operating of its own volition—but then again it is not my own voice that is speaking, it is that of someone else, although my own voice box is somehow forming the words.

Physically, you begin to feel "the other" building up internally. It is as if someone else is putting on your body from within. The arms, the legs, the hands adopt postures that are not characteristic of you. "You" may now abruptly get to "your" feet, as the he or she within you decides to stand up. Possibly then walking about the room, you experience the stiff joints and bent fingers of an arthritic, or the light, carefree limbs of a young girl. I am one of those individuals who remains conscious during trance—others black out completely—and I am always astonished when I hear "my" voice speaking with a pre-adolescent girl's tone, without any trace of falsetto or unnaturalness. The content of the spirits' speeches is also completely strange and new.

The reality of the physical concomitants of mediumship, then, need not be doubted. The question is, what exactly is happening? What is the basis of these astonishing events?

There are very many reasons for rejecting the idea that the spirits of the dead are involved. One is that the alleged spirits never tell us anything that is not already known to living persons on this planet—and, almost invariably, known to the bereaved person "sitting" with the medium.

The "spirits" tell us any amount of information known *only* to the sitter, which is why the session is often so very impressive for the sitter. Given this situation, the most likely explanation must be that the medium's unconscious mind is acquiring information paranormally from the mind of the sitter. (The sitter need not be consciously thinking about the matters in question, but they are nevertheless present somewhere in his or her mind.) That the medium possesses strong paranormal gifts cannot be doubted. What is being rejected here is the idea of involvement of discarnate spirits.

Anyone who studies the casebooks and autobiographies of the great mediums, such as Ena Twigg,[1] cannot fail to be impressed. In judging the material only two choices exist for the reader. Either the evidence from the sittings is genuine—or a monumental hoax has been perpetrated. Yet the second choice actually demands more credulity than the first.

Taking just one instance from Ena Twigg, Sir Victor Goddard, who had never visited a medium before, made an appointment with her. He told Ena only that he wished to contact a friend. She asked did he mean a big man, six foot two, and so forth, and went on then to give a full description of the person Goddard wanted to contact. In a subsequent session Ena went into trance. Goddard writes:

> Then she might sit back in her chair, her legs crossed and stretched out, and she might go through the motion of adjusting the eyeglass which Fawcett wore over his blind eye, a typical mannerism. She might use any of his mannerisms and his personal figures of speech. It wasn't so much the information which was conveyed as the manner of its conveying in speech, in action, and in gesture that carried conviction. . . .[2]

The real problem (for the spirit hypothesis) is that there is nothing in what the "spirits" narrate that persuades us that anything but a *memory* of that person is operating (taken, unconsciously, from the mind of the sitter by the medium). Would we not, for example, expect the spirit of a famous scientist or psychologist to *add* something to the knowledge and theories he left behind on earth. It does not—more of this aspect later. Neither do the spirit visitors convey anything of the delirious joy we might expect them to feel having wakened on "the other side," nor any convincing sense of actually being there. None of the descriptions given of the other side, always couched in the vaguest of generalizations, produces any impression of a real place. Without being unkind, naive is the only word to describe these accounts of the other world. Nor in any case do the various spirits, speaking within the frameworks of the various spiritist organizations, at all agree on the nature of the afterlife. A certain consensus is observed within any particular esoteric organization, but never between organizations. Compare, for example, the views of the Theosophists and the Spiritualists on the nature of the afterlife, the meaning of life on earth, and the purpose of the universe. Instances of the differences between groups follow.

Some of the visiting spirits speak at great length, and in fact dictate or write actual books. Two examples of such literary products are the famous *A Dweller on Two Planets* by "Phylos the Tibetan"[3] and the numerous "Seth" books written through Jane Roberts.

Frederick S. Oliver, an American, tells us that Phylos the Tibetan had "always" spoken to him inwardly. Then "when a little past seventeen years of age 'Phylos the Esoterist' took me actively in charge, designing to make me his instrument to the world. . . ." Oliver now became the amanuensis of this inner voice of his, which he considered to be a personification of the eternal Christ spirit, and *A Dweller on Two Planets* was published in 1886—under the authorship of Phylos the Tibetan since Oliver himself disclaimed all authorship. This is a rambling book, a kind of science fantasy or romance fantasy about Atlantis and how it once was, and the origins of man, involving Christ and a plethora of mythical and actual figures past and present. Even as a piece of occult fantasy or fiction the book seems very old-fashioned (and is nowhere near as good as, say, Michael Moorcock's novels); whereas Freud writing around the same time does not seem old-fashioned, any more than does Shakespeare writing some hundreds of years earlier. As objective truth, which is what the book purports to be, it is complete rubbish.

In case it seems a little unfair to pick on something written as long ago as 1886, let us take Jane Roberts, who is writing vigorously at the present time. Prior to her takeover by the "nonphysical energy personality essence" known as Seth, Roberts was a professional and prolific author, living with her artist husband. (Incidentally, Arthur Guirdham also used to write fiction.) When she was thirty-five Jane and her husband experimented more or less idly with a ouija board. The emergence of the Seth personality was the result. As in standard mediumship, Seth often takes over Jane Roberts completely, giving lectures and dispensing wisdom. He also dictates an apparently endless series of books to Jane, which she writes automatically in a form of trance.

A word on Jane Roberts's mediumship: In trance she undergoes the kind of dramatic facial, body, and personality changes already described. Photographs of her as herself, and in trance, show the expressions of two different personalities. As Seth, Jane Roberts becomes animated and eloquent, speaking in a deep, booming voice. The general character of Seth is quite unlike Jane's own. The mediumship itself is therefore genuine enough: that is, it partakes of that degree of spontaneous personality change that remains one of the unexplained wonders of the human psyche.

Yet what of the products of this mediumship? They are, alas, of the same level, though not the same type, of nonsense as that produced by Frederick Oliver. Here is an example of Seth's material.

> The structure of the psyche of the world at any given time can be ascertained by viewing its exterior condition: the various civilizations all representing actualized characteristics inherent in the world mind. The different governments act in response to inner politics, which are the result of multitudinous ones used by individuals in dealing with private inner and outer reality. . . .[4]

For myself, speaking as a professional psychologist, who is moreover very positive about the paranormal, these statements mean absolutely nothing. All of Seth's numerous books, in fact, mean absolutely nothing. (However, they sell by the million world-wide.)

Jane Roberts also receives communications from eminent psychologists and analysts like William James and C. G. Jung. Here is an example of Jung speaking.

> Numbers have an emotional equivalent, in that their symbols originally arose from the libido that always identifies itself with the number 1, and feels all other numbers originating out of itself. The libido knows itself as God, and therefore all fractions fly out of the self structure of its own reality. The Father-God and the physical father alike ally themselves with the number 1, and see their magical transformation occurring out of a constant addition, arising from their own basic omnipotence.
>
> The son, symbolized by 2, feels the father and the number 1 as a threat from which it emerges and from which the son emerges triumphant, grateful and yet rebelling. The 3 is the female principle, which neither the father nor son, nor 1 or 2, can deny.[5]

If this is really Jung, speaking from the other side, then he has gone bananas. How good it would be to be able to question this alleged Jung on some of the more abstruse points of his theories. I guarantee this Jung would not even understand the questions, let alone answer them. I doubt that if you gave him the titles of five of his papers he would be able to say in which order he had written them. (I once knew another medium who claimed that Jung spoke through her. I was not permitted to talk to this entity, but the medium played me some of the tape recordings. They were the same kind of high-sounding nonsense that we have just had.)

One notes in passing that the general views of Seth on the universe do not accord with those of Phylos the Tibetan, and neither accord with the views of mainstream Spiritualism. So who is right?

Interestingly, like Frederick Oliver, Jane Roberts admits to having had intimations of spirits most of her life. ". . . one way or another I get signals from strange lands. I always have, though when I was growing up I just labeled everything as inspiration and let it go at that. Finally inspiration had a voice of its own and a personage, Seth."

The interest lies in the fact that many artists of all kinds, though perhaps especially writers, feel that their source of inspiration is almost detached from them; it somehow seems to come to them from somewhere else, or someone else. (Mozart, for instance, felt that the music was not altogether of his making.) So the Greeks spoke of the Muses, actual goddesses who visited artists and philosophers to give them inspiration.

The Greeks also spoke of the "*daimon*" (our word "demon"), the active principle of a god that, similarly, visited and inspired human beings. Socrates had such a demon, to which he frequently referred. Artists, particularly romantic artists, have readily accepted these ideas. Even in common speech today we say "he painted like a man possessed." Indeed, the experience of writing furiously for days on end with little or no sleep or food does feel very much like an act of possession.

These points and this connection cannot be too strongly emphasized. So the writer Margaret Kennedy has the following passage in her novel *The Constant Nymph,* concerning the hero of the novel, Lewis, a composer. Tessa is a young friend, the daughter of another composer.

The thought so moved her that she flung herself down on the short wind-blown grass and gazed into the sky above her, waiting, in an effort to reach singleness of mind. Nothing happened. . . . Gazing now down towards the path Tessa saw that a man was standing there, staring at the mountains in a kind of lost trance, as if he had discovered the secret thing which had escaped her. It was Lewis. . . . Presently his vision seemed to break up, and he took to walking about, in a distraught frenzy, stumbling sometimes, and often almost running. She knew what ailed him and she was very sorry. Living in a family of artists she had come to regard this implacable thing which took them as a great misfortune. Oddly enough it had missed her out. She did not believe she would ever be driven to these monstrous creative efforts. . . . She pitied her friend when it assailed him as much as if he had fallen down and broken his leg. To her the thing was a hidden curse, a family werewolf, always ready to spring out and devour them all. It was at the bottom of most of their misfortunes. Its place in her scheme of things was approximate to the position which the devil might hold in the mind of a better instructed little girl.[6]

Intuitively, and as I would urge correctly, Margaret Kennedy firmly links the state of artistic and creative possession with the devil and the werewolf—with, in short, the state of demonic possession.

The artistic possessor and inspirer is, equally, not some discarnate entity, but one's own unconscious mind, temporarily shouldering aside normal consciousness in order to achieve its own ends. This view is further strongly supported by the fact that many artists find and acknowledge direct artistic inspiration in their own dreams. Robert Louis Stevenson, for example, dreamed the plot of his classic story of Jekyll and Hyde (and said that most of his literary inspiration came from dreams); and Coleridge composed "Kubla Khan" while dreaming, but woke up before it was finished. The choreographer, Lindsay Kemp, said in a recent interview that he usually gets his ideas for costumes from his dreams. There are very many examples.

Mediumship seems to be only an extreme and fully personified form of such unconscious overshadowing. (We ought to note in passing that it is the nature of the unconscious mind to produce a myriad personalities, which it throws off endlessly, perhaps as a kind of smokescreen to hide its true nature; whereas the conscious mind itself possesses only one personality.) Mediums, however, also have full access to the paranormal abilities of the unconscious mind, which the artist taps only very occasionally. (Chapter 16, however, discusses some instances of the artist as psychic.)

As we have seen, many people produce automatic writing without any suggestion of the presence of discarnate spirits—it can be readily induced by hypnosis, for example (see chapter 5). Anita Mühl's patients produced very "inspirational" automatic scripts, but again without spirits being involved.

The fact is that all and any of the phenomena of mediumship can be produced by people who are not mediums, and, moreover, in circumstances where we have no need whatsoever to invoke the theory of discarnate entities as an explanation. In particular, all the impressive features of so-called spirit possession are produced in hypnotic regression, and in the clinical condition of multiple personality.

Mediumship is in itself a genuine phenomenon. The sad fact is, however, that as long as mediums and other automatists claim to be in contact with departed spirits, orthodox science and academic psychology will continue to have an excuse to dismiss all the phenomena involved as nonsense. As a result this marvel of the human mind will continue to go unrecorded and undiscussed in the textbooks of our universities.

In conclusion, we must note that a majority of mediums are female. C. D. Broad remarks "most eminent trance mediums in western countries for the past 150 years have been women,"[7] and the list of sensitives recommended at the time of writing by the College of Psychic Studies in London comprises eleven women and one man. How is it that the alleged spirits of the dead communicate more easily with females than males? Sadly again, such pertinent questions are seldom asked by Spiritualists. This particular question is perhaps all the more intriguing when we consider that women are banned from office in many Western and Middle Eastern religions—in fact in virtually all religions worldwide.

10

DISCARNATES?

A significant point in the argument against so-called discarnate or spirit entities having any separate, independent existence is the encounter with the "ghosts" of those still very much alive. This event occurs quite frequently and strikingly. These non-ghost ghostly encounters do not, of course, by themselves prove that the dead do not return as spirits, or the nonexistence of discarnate spirits of non-human origin (that is, demons or angels). But in respect of human ghosts at least, such encounters hit the ball firmly into the survivalists' court. Believers in spirits must prove a difference between the "ghosts" of those who are very much still alive and the alleged returning spirits of those who have died. Just to claim a difference will not do at all.

The poet W. B. Yeats, for example, reports an incident where he sat down to write a note to a student many tens of miles away that was vital to the student's future. At this point, though he did not know Yeats was writing to him, the student clearly saw Yeats in a crowd of people in a hotel, and again later that night when alone in his room.[1] The German poet and scientist, Goethe, also reports a striking "visitation." While out for a walk in the country, on a lonely road, a friend appeared momentarily before him whom he had not seen or contacted for many years. When Goethe arrived home he found the friend sitting waiting for him, perfectly well, and on a surprise visit.[2]

In pursuit of the policy of concentrating on the present day however, we turn to current cases. One incident comes from journalist Ted Simon, writing in the London *Times* of 3 January 1983. Simon, accompanied by his wife and son, called on a widowed friend of his mother's in Essex one rainy afternoon. The house lights were on. After ringing the bell several times, Simon looked through the window and saw the woman concerned walk from her kitchen and across the living room toward the front door. "Here she comes," said Simon to his family. He adds that she was back-lit by the kitchen light, so he could not see her face clearly. "But she was solid enough otherwise and I recognized her distinctive gait."

The woman failed to appear at the front door, and the visitors assumed she must have popped upstairs. Several times more they rang in vain. Returning now to his mother's house nearby, Simon telephoned the woman, thinking perhaps the doorbell might be out of order. There was no reply. He went back to the woman's house in some puzzlement. Looking through the window again, he now saw the woman going back through her kitchen door, the light making a halo of her characteristically fluffed-out hairstyle. Answer the doorbell, however, she did not.

The next day Simon telephoned the woman and spoke to her. She was perfectly well and had been away from home all day Sunday but had left the house lights on as usual, to deter burglars.[3]

Examples of these brief encounters could be multiplied, but instead we shall shortly consider a prolonged and very striking case of a "haunting" by the "ghost" of a very vigorously living person. First, a case of haunting by a person who never existed in the first place. The incident in question was set up as an experiment in connection with Colin Wilson's television series "Leap in the Dark" in the late 1970s. A writer, Frank Smythe, deliberately put round an entirely fictitious story that a particular place was haunted by a particular ghost. No one, apart from Smythe and the team, knew that the story was fictitious. A while later the researchers were *flooded* with reports from people claiming to have sighted the ghost in question. In this case, then, we have sightings of a ghost that arose simply on the basis of the public suggestion that there was a ghost to be seen. Is this not exactly what happens in respect of most well-known haunted locations? (Once again we seem to have an example of the process we have already observed, and will continue to observe, in other contexts, namely "you see what you expect to see/you see what you want to see.")

However, it is possibly not the case that every single person who sees a well-known ghost has had prior warning of that ghost's existence. In such cases we might argue that they had picked up the information telepathically from those who do know. Yet some, no doubt, knew of the ghost unconsciously, even though they had consciously forgotten about it (see chapters 6 and 7 on such "forgotten" material). We are then not a thousand miles either from the woman who saw a ghost as a result of a post-hypnotic command, again one of the experiments conducted by "Leap in the Dark." In the present chapter we have a further reminder that the unconscious mind forgets nothing.

The sighting of a ghost of a person at the moment of, or just after, or just before that person's death is very common, and there is no doubt at all that the *fact* of the death is somehow being communicated paranormally to the viewer of the ghost at that moment. (The "ghost" seen just before death nevertheless presents problems for the survivalist view—since, after all, the person concerned is not yet dead and is, in some cases at least, still very much in his or her own body.) Those interested in past instances of this phenomenon can glut themselves on Gurney, Myers and Podmore's *Phantasms of the Living*[4] or Eleanor Sidgwick's identically titled *Phantasms of the Living*.[5] There are many examples, too, of animal pets reacting to the death of their distant owners and of owners reacting to the death of distant pets, and a number of cases, both past and present, are cited in an earlier book of my own.[6]

Two "moment of death" visitations come from the famous medium of the last century, D. D. Home. At the age of thirteen, living in Troy, New York, and while getting ready for bed one evening, he had a glowing vision of his friend Edwin, then living in Greenville, Connecticut, a distance of many miles. Home told members of his family, "I have seen Edwin—he died three days ago." Two days after that came the news that Edwin had died unexpectedly after a short illness. At a later date Home suddenly cried out in the presence of others. He told the family that his mother (staying with friends a considerable distance away) had died at twelve o'clock midday, because "he had seen her and she had told him." Home's claim proved accurate.[7]

Let us now take two present-day examples from the case of Ruth, which is discussed later in this chapter in detail. Ruth was a psychiatric patient who produced remarkable hallucinations, sometimes with paranormal aspects. During an experimental session with her psychiatrist, Dr. Morton Schatzman, Ruth was asked to hallucinate a figure and to talk to it, to see if the replies of the apparition would make any impression on a tape recorder (they didn't). However, a figure materialized to Ruth before she had a chance to tell her mind to produce one. It was her grandmother. The apparition of the grandmother said that she was waiting for Ruth at home (the grandmother was in America, and Ruth in London—Ruth was supposed to visit soon). Then the apparition said: "No matter what happens, you'll always have me. I don't want you to worry that you won't." Ruth then asked: "Will I ever see you? Will you be dead when I get home?" To which the grandmother answered: "I'll only be as dead as you'll let me be. Hold your head up, you're as good as the best and better than the rest." As the grandmother spoke these words she had tears running down her face and was smiling.

That incident occurred at 4:30 P.M. The grandmother in America in fact died the same day at 11 P.M. London time, six and a half hours later.

Ruth's father and the father's mother and brother also experienced a "vision of death." Ruth's father's sister, Debbie, had become a drug addict, and to support the habit had turned to prostitution. For this she had been banned from the house and forbidden to return. At this time Debbie was only seventeen years old. One day, sitting on the porch, the father, his brother, and his mother saw a horse and carriage draw up in the street in front of the house. Debbie got out and walked up to the wooden gate. She did not open it. She looked very ill. Then she walked away down the street. Just after Debbie had gone, a policeman came to the house to say that Debbie had just died in hospital from an overdose.[8]

This kind of case is among the strongest evidence for the view of a detachable spirit that survives the death of the human body. The family was not expecting Debbie's death—they did not even know she was in the hospital. The vision was seen by three different people simultaneously. And the visitation occurred very shortly *after* death. The "surviving spirit" explanation here is no wilder than the non-spirit alternative—which has to involve, in this particular case, not just telepathic communication of the fact of death, but also a detailed, collective hallucination, a rather rare event in itself. (We might, perhaps, point out the "suspicious" circumstances that the spirit was nevertheless dancing to the family's tune. *They* had forbidden her to come to the house, and even in death she went on obeying them. She was doing what they would have expected her to do in reality. Why did she not come up to them, and smile her forgiveness, or ask their forgiveness?)

When large numbers of hauntings are analyzed we find 84 percent to be visual, 37 percent auditory, 15 percent involve touch, and 8 percent smell.[9] These various amounts of sensory impression just happen to reflect rather closely the degree of importance that each of these senses plays in our normal lives, and is catered for in the sensory cortex of the brain. It can certainly be argued that the spirit visitor is necessarily manipulating *our* nervous system, so that such results might be expected. But a less demanding explanation is that it is our own nervous system that is producing the phenomenon in the first place, and so the phenomenon bears its stamp.

The spirit hypothesis works much less well in many other examples. Mentioned earlier was the fact that animals react to the distant death of their owners, and owners to the distant death of their pets. An instance of the latter is reported (from 1924) regarding a Mr. Grindle Matthews. Matthews, a London engineer, was in New York on business. One early morning he woke sweating profusely from a nightmare in which he had seen his pet cat struggling in the hands of a man with a goatee beard wearing a white coat. The hotel room seemed to Matthews to reek of chloroform, and the smell of it haunted him for days afterwards. He told others of these circumstances. It was later established that the housekeeper in London had had the cat put down at the moment when Matthews had his nightmare, and that the vet (not known to Matthews) had had a goatee beard.[10]

We can, if we wish, assume that cats and other animals have souls and that the dying or discarnate cat had somehow produced Matthew's nightmare. However, a telepathic rapport between the two organisms is an equally good explanation here—and in many other cases is the only possible explanation. These other numerous cases, attested to by vets and other witnesses of standing show that some pets (whether boarded in kennels or not) exhibit unmistakable signs of delirious joy at the moment when their absent owners set out from a distant location to return home.[11] Dogs will dash upstairs and bring the master's slippers, and place them by the fire, for example, meanwhile leaping about and wagging their tails in transports of joy. Pet animals likewise respond appropriately when their distant owners are in any danger. There are many authenticated cases of all kinds of animals—cats, horses, dogs, and so on—who have tracked their owners, sometimes across *thousands* of miles of unknown country. Beyond any doubt, the owner is transmitting some kind of message, some kind of homing signal, which the animal is able to follow.

In all these cases we do not require the discarnate spirit hypothesis at all. It is totally irrelevant. Why, then, do we need it as an explanation when a close friend or relative happens to have a vision of a dead or dying person? (As emphasized, the person is not always dead when the vision occurs.) Is it not enough to say in all cases of death that having received some kind of telepathic impulse of events, the unconscious mind then generates some kind of symbolic fantasy—a vision, a dream, a premonition—by which means it presents the received information to consciousness?

That view gains enormously also from the fact that Australian aborigines are very good at sensing the death of a distant companion. But they do not see a ghostly vision of that person, as westerners often do. Instead they see a vision of that person's totem animal running about the camp.[12] Once again, "we see what we expect to see" in terms of our cultural (and in this case religious) upbringing. The totem animal is the best choice, and the obvious choice, for the Aborigine unconscious mind to make in presenting its information to consciousness.

Finally, before moving on to consider the case of Ruth in detail, we should mention a study of hallucinations of the bereaved. W. Demi Rees[13] asked 293 surviving husbands and wives (66 men, 227 women) whether they had ever "felt the presence of, seen, heard, been spoken to or touched by" the dead spouse. Almost half (46.7 percent) said they had. Perhaps the most interesting finding of this study was that young people, that is, those below the age of forty, were much less likely to hallucinate than those over forty—21 percent of the former as opposed to 50 percent of the latter. The hallucinations were particularly strong in those over sixty. Now, is it the case that the dead communicate more easily or readily with the elderly (it could be argued that older people need this spiritual comfort more than younger people)? Or is it rather that the older and lonelier one is, the more likely the unconscious mind is to generate phantasms of the departed? We know from life as well as from many experiments that both social and sensory deprivation are conducive to the production of hallucinations. Hermits often have them, for example. The fact is that man is a social animal, to the very depths of his being. Starved of the real thing, he tends to generate ghostly companions of his own.

The small study just cited needs repeating with much larger groups—but one other of its results deserves mention, namely that slightly more men than women experienced the dead partner (50 percent of the men as opposed to 45.8 percent of the women). This is an unexpected finding, in view of what we know about mediumship (see chapter 9) and hallucinations generally. In the Society for Psychical Research's investigation into "Spontaneous Hallucinations of the Sane," for example, when 8372 men and 8628 women were interviewed, 12 percent of the women as opposed to 8 percent of the men admitted to having had a "vivid, spontaneous hallucination" at some point in their lives.[14]

We come now to psychiatrist Morton Schatzman's book *The Story of Ruth*,[15] a case study of a remarkable woman. As a child in America Ruth had had a very vivid relationship with her dolls, to whom she talked and who talked to her. She also saw full, vivid apparitions (such as "a man in white")—the first shortly before her fourth birthday—which continued intermittently throughout her life. Many children display the doll behavior, of course, but Ruth's was of an intensity and duration that produced rebukes from her mother and mockery from her brothers and sisters, and in therapy Ruth recalled her deep unhappiness at this treatment. This material is of general interest when we come later to "the natural history of the psychic." It is also of particular interest both here and then in respect to neurosis (see chapters 13 and 14), where it seems that the rejection—by parents and other siblings—of a burgeoning psychic gift may result in unpleasant or uncontrolled paranormal events in later life. What is being suggested here, and to use the terminology of depth psychology, is that the psychic aspects of the personality are repressed or disowned in childhood and then, like repressed sexuality and repressed aggression, lead to severe personality problems in later life—of which those experienced by Ruth are perhaps an example.

At any rate, at the age of twenty-five, and now living in London with her husband, Ruth sought psychiatric help. She was suffering from very severe and rather unusual neurotic symptoms. She was, in point of fact, extremely lucky to chance upon an enlightened psychiatrist like Schatzman, for otherwise she might easily have found herself hospitalized as a diagnosed schizophrenic.

Some of Ruth's presenting symptoms were as follows. She had developed an aversion to sex with her husband and now found this disgusting. She had also taken to keeping all the doors in the house locked and trembled if she had to open the front door. She was afraid of crowds, public places, and doors of all kinds, both open and closed. She feared being in enclosed and constricting places as much as she feared being in the open. She spent all day crying and had no appetite for food. She felt depressed and guilty about her condition and about neglecting her home and children, a circumstance that in turn led to more guilt and depression. She now feared in particular that her brain was going to explode. So great was the sense of internal pressure that she believed that the skull would rupture.

She also had troubled, repetitive nightmares. She would dream that she woke up. A numb, tingling feeling would spread, rising, through her body. Her tongue would become thick and heavy. Then, when she began to speak, blood would spatter from her mouth all over the ceiling and walls. These dreams were becoming stronger and more frequent.

It transpired that when she was ten, Ruth had been the victim of a rape by her father. He had come into her room one night when drunk. In a prolonged session he had tried to have intercourse with her—normally, orally, and anally. All these attempts had failed, both because of her smallness and her resistance. In the course of them he punched her heavily and bit her nipples till they bled. (She still bears the scars of these bites.) Finally he masturbated into Ruth's hair and left telling her that he would kill her if she told anyone what had happened. She did, however, tell her mother, who also said she must keep silent—otherwise her father would go to prison. (Years later, when Ruth had married, her father spoke suggestively to her about the rape experience, and on a later occasion he fondled her, told her he had always been and still was sexually attracted to her, and wanted to make love to her. There was, apparently, a strong history of incest in the family.)

Ruth now reported another recurrent dream to the psychiatrist. She is ten years old again, and her father comes into the room and has full sexual intercourse with her. Blood spurts out of her vagina. When she wakes up, in reality that is, she looks at her husband Paul. He has become her father. Thereafter, by day, Paul sometimes turns into her father. She also now dreams that Paul rapes her.

Before proceeding with the narration, an extremely important point must be made. *If* Ruth's father had now been dead, the events that follow would undoubtedly have been ascribed by occultists and spiritualists to the activities of the dead man's spirit. He is, they would have said, earthbound because of his evil. He cannot rise to the proper levels of spirit. So great is his evil, indeed, that he wants to go on perpetrating his wickedness now that he is dead, and his discarnate situation gives him the opportunity for this.

The foregoing is, *without any doubt at all*, the "explanation" that would have been put forward. It *is* continually put forward in such cases. But Ruth's father was not dead; he was alive and perfectly well in America.

Prior to Ruth attending for therapy, her father had begun appearing, independently, all over the house at all times. It was as if he were actually living there. These apparitions were totally real to Ruth. They engaged all the senses: sight, sound (she heard not just his voice, but footsteps and so on), smell, touch, movement. When he shook the bed she felt it move. When he squeezed her hand it hurt. When he opened the bathroom door on her she felt a draught. Upstairs, she would hear him close the living-room door downstairs and go out, but no one else could see or hear him. The intentions of the apparition were twofold—to have intercourse with Ruth and to persecute her to death.

Clearly, the apparition of Ruth's father was behaving like an incubus and possessed its powers. Later, Ruth did have actual sexual intercourse with one of her apparitions—not her father, but an apparition of her husband, Paul.

In her sixth session with Schatzman Ruth's father materialized in the consulting room. Schatzman reports that Ruth was absolutely terrified. "I have never seen anyone so overcome by fear."

In Schatzman's view, no separate entity was involved, only some aspect of Ruth's unconscious mind. His therapeutic efforts therefore centered on getting Ruth to accept that she herself was producing the, apparently, totally unwelcome visitor, and that since she was producing the apparition, she could also control it. She was persecuting herself—the tail, so to speak, was wagging the dog. Despite an initial worsening of symptoms (the father now followed her in the street and accompanied her on tube trains), Schatzman eventually succeeded in giving Ruth the courage to face the apparition, before which she had initially fled in terror:

She had wakened in the morning to see her father sitting at her dressing table, a toothpick in his mouth. She had decided to be bold with him.

"What do you want?" she asked him as she lay in bed.

"You know what I want," he said.

She tried to be strong. "I don't care if you stay here. I'm not going to be bothered."

"I don't care what you say," he replied. "When I leave you I do so because I want to, not because you tell me to."

He started to approach her bed as he said it.

She jumped out of bed, put on a dressing gown and ran out of the room.[16]

When the father began appearing in the consulting room Schatzman was able to talk to him through Ruth. She relayed the replies, which only she heard. This device was extremely useful therapeutically. Sometimes Schatzman went to sit in the chair occupied by Ruth's father—at which point the father beat a hasty retreat. Occasionally Ruth saw Dr. Schatzman as her father, and Schatzman encouraged her to experiment. At one point she produced two Schatzmans. Ruth was beginning to realize that she *could* control her apparitions. She began hallucinating a great friend of hers, Becky, with whom she was then able to have long and comforting conversations. (It is important to realize that Ruth did not know in advance how an apparition would behave: its freedom of action was that of a normal person—though, as with a normal visitor, she could relate to it, ask it to do things, persuade it, confront it, and so on.) The real Becky, of course, was—like Ruth's father—still very much alive in America. Then Ruth succeeded in producing an apparition of herself (which she found very disturbing), an important feature of a later event.

Aspects of Ruth's apparitions closely resemble the phenomena of multiple personality. Sometimes Ruth would feel she *was* the apparition, for a little while at least. Then, as Ruth, that is as her real self, she would have a memory blank (amnesia) in respect of herself for that interval. Ruth could touch her apparitions as well as be touched by them. They felt entirely physically real to her.

Now we move even further toward the events of the typical spiritualist séance. Ruth had discovered that she could make her own face in the mirror turn into her father's face, and then get it to talk. (Miss Beauchamp in chapter 14 accidentally hit upon just the same device of the mirror, except that the "possessor" wrote its communications, using her own hand in automatic writing.) Here we have a situation that very closely parallels the possession of the entranced medium by a discarnate spirit. Subsequently, a complete parallel developed.

Schatzman, standing behind Ruth while she looked in the mirror, was now able to converse directly with the father. The father, still completely self-willed, discussed his own view of the rape, and many other aspects of his own life and thought. Then, a little later, Ruth was able to go into trance without the mirror and "become" her father. An intriguing point is that while the father was discussing his own sexual arousal over the rape, and also over his own sister, Debbie, the real Ruth (observing and listening within herself, as many mediums do) became sexually aroused herself. These direct interviews with Ruth's father are really quite extraordinary. There is all the vividness of speech and thought patterns of another, entirely different, personality. This material is every bit the equal of the products of the best trance mediums.

But Ruth's father was not dead. There was no discarnate spirit. Is there *ever* a discarnate spirit in a séance room? Almost certainly not.

These trance sessions left Ruth physically dazed and shaken. How easy it *would have been* (both for her and us) to believe that she had been taken over by a violent, earth-bound spirit. Schatzman remarks: "When her 'father' was speaking, Ruth's face seemed expressionless, mask-like and stiff in a way that I found uncharacteristic of her." (We shall have noted these facial and bodily changes in many different, or allegedly different, contexts by the end of this book.) In these sessions, incidentally, Ruth recalled many details of her life as a child that she had consciously completely forgotten.

We can leave the fine detail of Ruth's story at this point—her therapy, finally, ended happily—but there are three more items of value to summarize.

The first is that Ruth twice made love with an apparition of her husband Paul, which she deliberately created for that specific purpose. "He kissed my mouth again. Then he began to make love to me. I had my arms round him and could feel his back. . . . We climaxed together. As he came I felt his penis contract inside me, and heard him moan."

Schatzman asked her how satisfying the experience was sexually. She replied that it was very satisfying and that the apparition would be a good substitute for Paul whenever he was away. (One must stress again that the incubus-succubus *is* a very good substitute.)

Here, certainly, we *are* talking about an incubus. It is not the full *poltergeist*–incubus, for there is no record of any paranormal movement or breaking of objects in Ruth's story. However, there is evidence that others could see Ruth's apparitions on occasion. And there is also solid evidence from laboratory experiments with Ruth that her experiences were something more than "just" imagination. These items now follow.

During her therapy, when she was feeling considerably better, Ruth went home to America for a visit to her family, without Paul. She felt strong enough to face her father (who, of course, knew nothing that had been taking place in Ruth's life concerning his own apparition). One day she was walking down the road with her father back to their car. As they drew near it, Ruth placed a hallucination of Paul behind the steering wheel. Then she told her father to look at the car, because it looked as if there was someone in it. Her father said: "Oh, yeah. It looks like a ghost sitting there. Isn't that the damndest thing? It looks like a man, just like Paul." Then, on a later occasion, when Paul and Ruth were both together in America, Ruth had made an apparition of herself, sitting on the sofa, to ask it whether the plane in which she, Ruth, was returning to England would crash. Paul was in the kitchen next door, and now came in. When he saw Ruth sitting in her chair by the door he did a double-take. How could she be sitting in the chair, when he had seen her sitting on the sofa as he came into the room? Ruth asked him how the apparition of her had been sitting—with its feet tucked under it, was the reply. That was how Ruth had also seen her apparition. Were these cases of telepathy? Or had Ruth's visions achieved a momentary objective existence?

A number of laboratory experiments with Ruth were conducted in London by Dr. Schatzman once Ruth's therapy had been completed. She had lost none of her ability to hallucinate, but it was now under her control. Without going into the details of all the experiments, what Schatzman and his colleagues established was that when one of Ruth's apparitions put its hands over her eyes, or when it passed between her and a light source, what is known as the visual evoked response in Ruth's brain (monitored by electrodes) dropped sharply—just as it does when a *real* person does these things to us. Yet we have no control over the electrical emissions of our brains in any direct sense—we cannot influence these matters consciously. The same finding was established for sound: when Ruth had one of her hallucinations go over and turn down the volume on a machine emitting measured sounds, her auditory evoked response disappeared completely—although the real machine continued to emit noise! Finally, when Ruth caused a hallucinated figure to dab her arm with hallucinated cotton wool dipped in methylated spirits, the fine hairs on that spot on the back of her arm became erect as they do on a human arm when real methylated spirits is applied.

These experiments and others take Ruth's hallucinated figures well beyond any effect one can achieve by using one's normal imagination. Ruth's hallucinations here take a definite step toward objective existence. That is to say, these experimentally verified events blur, or move the position of, the line between subjective and objective reality. A further movement of that line also occurs when the extreme phenomena of multiple personality are examined. Here the alternative persona, when in residence, produces its own, distinctive brain electroencephalogram patterns (chapter 14). This is a change of *style* that we can in no way produce ourselves.

As always, we cannot finally prove that there is no such thing as a discarnate entity. What we can show, in more and more contexts, is that there is a better and simpler explanation, involving far fewer assumptions, than the theory of discarnates. We succeed, simultaneously, in bringing the alleged entity more under developmental and investigative control, both on our own account and experimentally. The concept of the haunted person, in particular, enables us to see an individual spinning a universe of strange events out of thin air, events that include apparent discarnates. But the alleged discarnates do not *produce* the phenomena, as is often incorrectly claimed. They themselves are simply *part* of the phenomena. The concept of the haunted individual can be extended to the concept of the haunted family. That is, psychic individuals tend to run in families—there is a genetic, inherited component also. Thus Ruth's aunt Grace used to hallucinate and talk to her husband after his death, and Ruth's son George has an invisible companion called Georgie. As we saw too, Ruth's father and others in her blood family also possessed telepathic abilities.

In conclusion, it is very much worth emphasizing that the events of the second half of this chapter occurred in modern London, in the late 1970s. But roll back the clock a hundred years, and Ruth would have been sitting not in a doctor's surgery, but in a séance room. And back another four hundred she would have been strapped in the Inquisitor's chair, before being burned.

11

LEFT-HANDEDNESS

The Maoris of New Zealand believe that "the right is the side of the gods, where hovers the white figure of a good guardian angel; the left side is dedicated to demons or to the devil, and a black and wicked angel holds it in dominion."[1] On the other side of the world, in the northern hemisphere, and in a totally different time-and-space capsule, Muslims believe that both prophets and diviners are inspired by familiars; but whereas the former, who wear white, hear the words of their invisible companions at their right ear, the latter, who wear black, receive their instruction in the left ear.[2] There is no coincidence involved here. Precisely the same divisions and attitudes are found in every single nation in the world. They form part of the growing body of evidence that the religious and legendary folk material of every single people is traceable back to one common source; a scarcely believable circumstance, and yet true.[3]

Our primary concern here, however, is with the universal division of events into left-sided and right-sided, and with the implications of that situation for our arguments.

"The power of the left hand is always occult and illegitimate, it inspires terror and revulsion. . . . Beings which are believed to possess dreadful magical powers are represented as left-handed"[4] (Thus in medieval Europe the raised devil is habitually shown stepping from the magic pentagram with left hand outstretched.) Most intriguingly, the further universal emphasis is that the *left* is *female*. This is a most odd view in any normal reasoning, since there are fewer left-handed females than males in the general population—a situation that pertains throughout the world, even among the Chinese for instance, where a recent large-scale, careful study reports the incidence of left-handedness to be double that found in the West.[5]

In a brief global review, and in no particular order, we find that the Maoris consider the right hand to be male and active, the left to be female and passive.[6] Further, right for them represents life and left represents death. Among the North American Indians the right similarly represents bravery and virility, and the left death and burial.[7] In China, as soon as children are capable of picking up food, they *must* be taught to eat with the right hand.[8] In the Dutch Indies the local native populations bind the left hand of the child, to teach him or her not to use it.[9] Actual mutilation of the left arm is found in a number of societies in the world,[10] and the Nuer peoples of Africa also bind the left arm with metal rings to put it out of action "for long periods."[11]

Distributed throughout the African continent, as among the ancient Arab peoples, are the views (a) that the left is female, and the right male, and (b) that the right signifies good and the left evil.[12] Men are habitually buried lying on their right side, and women lying on the left side. In some tribes women are not allowed to use the left hand while cooking, and in others they must never touch the husband's face with the left hand.

These habits and attitudes are duplicated also in South America. There, as ever, the right is good and the left evil, the right is life and the left is death, the right is the man, and the left the woman-child.[13]

Of great interest too are the views spread throughout all Indonesian peoples concerning the precise relationship of death and left-handedness. (Some African tribes also echo something of these views.) The Ngaja of southern Borneo say that language reverses in afterlife—right becomes left, straight becomes crooked, sweet becomes bitter, and so on. The Toraja of Celebes also believe that the dead use words with opposite meaning (yes means no, and so on), and also pronounce them backwards. The Batak of Sumatra say that the dead reverse everything—they walk backwards, go about by night instead of day, and so on. But the Toraja go still farther. They say that the face, the feet and the chest of the dead are turned backwards.[14]

We know (chapter 2) that the feet of the night hag Lilith are also turned backwards, as is the head of the Chinese vampire. Our own European vampire also indulges in reversals, of course. He lives by night and sleeps by day.

Perhaps more significantly still, many people who produce automatic writing in trance and under hypnosis (chapter 5) also sometimes write backwards and, where both hands are employed simultaneously, the left produces a different narrative from the right. Most of the ancient peoples and some of the modern peoples we are discussing could not write at all. But they could draw. Did the mediums of these nations, in trance, draw backwards, or use the left hand in preference to the right? Did they, perhaps, *speak backwards?* We have no records in current times of mediums speaking backwards—but since to write backwards is no problem at all, there seems no reason in principle to rule out the speaking achievement. It is, at any rate, most interesting that the Lord's Prayer and other items of the Black Mass are spoken backwards.

There are further probably significant links in this chain. Children suffering from dyslexia (word-blindness) often write individual letters backwards. The neuropsychologist R. Llinas has recently shown that the individual character of our handwriting is conferred by that part of the brain called the cerebellum.[15] A much earlier study had demonstrated that 97 percent of a random sample of those suffering from dyslexia also showed cerebellar-vestibular dysfunction.[16] As it happens, the cerebellum itself is left-handed in relation to the main brain. (These matters are discussed in detail in chapter 17.)

Women have larger cerebella than men,[17] and among ancient peoples, as in the modern west, more women were trance mediums than men (see chapter 9). Is the cerebellum perhaps responsible both for trance itself and for left-handedness, and for the behavior reversals seen in trance?

Moving toward the European tradition, in India the right and the left are, again, clearly identified with the male and female respectively.[18] "The clearest statement of this association of sides with sexuality is the frequent iconographic representation of Siva as Ardhanarisvara . . . the right side of the figure has the hip, shoulder and chest of a man, while the left side is fashioned with the thigh, waist, and breast of a woman."

In the Greek tradition the right–left, male–female, light–dark paired connections are set out in the Pythagorean Table of Opposites, as reported by Aristotle; and Anaxagoras considered that the left testicle was responsible for female children and the right testicle for male babies. The left is universally unlucky in the classical world.[19]

In the Koran, the elect are on the right of the Lord and the damned on his left. In the Muslim tradition "God struck Adam's back and drew forth from him all his progeny. The men predestined for heaven came forth from the right side in the form of pearl-like white grain; those doomed to hell came forth from the left side in the form of charcoal-like black grain."[20] The writer Tabori states: "Allah has nothing left-handed about him, since both his hands are right hands."[21]

Similarly, in the Christian tradition, "it is not by chance that in pictures of the Last Judgment it is the Lord's raised right hand that indicates to the elect their sublime abode, while his lowered left hand shows the damned the gaping jaws of hell ready to swallow them."[22] Also "Christian saints in the cradle were so pious as to refuse the left breast of their mothers."

Ignoring such further "trivial" matters as the fact that in Europe the male buttons his coat toward the right, while the female buttons hers toward the left, we turn instead to a consideration of philology.

In the vast Indo-European family of languages (which embraces the Indian subcontinent, various Middle Eastern languages such as Iranian and Hittite, as well as Russian, Greek, Latin, German, French, Celtic, and so on) the words for "right" are very few, and persist from the earliest historical times. Thus the English word "right" is reflected in German *recht,* French *droit,* and so on; and the root *deks* (from which we have our word "dexterous" = skillful, from the Latin *dexter* = on the right hand) occurs also in Indo-Iranian, Celtic, Lithuanian, Slavonic, Albanian, Germanic, and elsewhere.

By complete contrast all Indo-European languages have a different word for left—for example, French *gauche,* Italian *mancino,* Latin *sinister.* Indeed, it seems to be the case that every dialect in every language has its own word for left, and left-handedness generates endless nicknames, which right-handedness never acquires. In English some of these have crept into the standard language: cack-handed, bollock-handed, coochy, squiffy, wacky, southpaw, cowpaw, and so on. The standard word for left also always means something totally derogatory. "Left" itself (from Old English *lyft*) means "weak, worthless, womanish," Italian *mancino* means "dubious, dishonest," French *gauche* means "awkward," Latin *sinister* is English "sinister" (and has this meaning also in Latin), and so on. The practice appears to hold outside Europe also: among the Nyoro in Africa, for example, "left" means "hated," and in Japan *hiddarimaki* means "crazy."

Nor is this by any means all. The words for "right" in the Indo-European languages spawn all kinds of other excellent words based on it: from "right" we have direct, erect, erection, correct, rectitude, rector, regal, royal, regime, regiment, rights, forthright, upright, and so on. From *deks,* apart from dexterous, we have dignity, decent, decree, doctrine, decorum, and so forth. Here we see nothing less than a profile of the authoritarian personality. The many words for left in the Indo-European languages, by contrast, produce *no derivatives whatsoever.* Might the left personality profile, if it existed, be that of the non-authoritarian, female personality?

The active persecution continues in many parts of the modern world today. In Italy, for example, left-handedness "is regarded as a personal and moral defect," and the most strenuous efforts are made to "correct" it.[23] In Japan left-handers are still automatically corrected—but "enlightenment" has reached the point where teachers now first ask parents whether they have any objection to the "correction" being undertaken.[24] ("Correct," of course, is itself one of the words derived from "right.") A still worse position pertains in modern Taiwan (see below).

In Britain we are just beginning to see the effects of a more liberal education system that no longer attempts to impose handedness on children, but allows them to make their own natural choice. When Cyril Burt examined a sample of 5,000 English elementary schoolchildren in 1937 he reported 5.8 percent of the boys to be left-handed and 3.7 percent of the girls (average 4.8 percent).[25] In 1959 Margaret Clark examined 72,238 Scottish schoolchildren of all categories and found 6.68 percent of the boys to be left-handed, as opposed to 4.41 percent of the girls (average 5.56 percent).[26] Then in 1976 the National Child Development Study reported its findings on a random sample of 11,000 seven-year-olds throughout Britain. Here the figures are boys: 11.3 percent and girls: 8.8 percent (average 10 percent).[27]

What a remarkable and illustrative picture this is. While the groups concerned are not totally comparable in every respect, what we see is an average "increase" in left-handedness from 4.8 percent in 1937, through 5.56 percent in 1959, to 10 percent in 1976. Have we seen the upper limits of left-handedness yet? Probably not. Most interestingly, the gap between boys and girls does not appear to be narrowing. There is just a chance that girls are both subject to more pressure to conform than boys, and indeed accept that pressure more readily, so that further liberalization might see the incidence gap between the sexes narrowing—but this seems unlikely. However, Burt remarks that "the sex-difference tends definitely to diminish with age"—so we had better not be too dogmatic.

There are many problems in all this material, both for ourselves and for orthodoxy. First, how does orthodoxy account for the universal association between the left hand and the female, when it is persistently clear that there is actually a higher incidence of left-handedness among men? Second, how is it that "a slight difference of degree in the physical strength of the two hands" should become the focus for a division of the total universe into good and evil—an absolutely central and worldwide focus? Third, how is it these same attitudes and taboos still persist today in our so-called rational age? It is to the proof of this third claim that we now turn.

The vast majority of psychology and physiology textbooks today contain no reference to the subject of left-handedness. (We find precisely the same silence here as we find on the subject of the cerebellum—see chapter 17.) Anyone can check the truth of this statement for himself or herself. How is it that a topic that has centrally exercised the mind of man for thousands of years has suddenly ceased to exist? The answer is that it has not—witness the current taboos in Italy, Japan, and China, for example—although there is better grist for our mill than that. What has happened is that the subject of the significance of the left hand has been dropped: it has been censored.

The very occasional references to left-handedness that one does find are of two kinds: (1) those in the context of handicap and (2) those in the context of the "division of labor" between the two cerebral hemispheres of the main brain.

Taking the second point first—and we must remember that the left so-called major cerebral hemisphere governs the right of the body, and the right so-called minor hemisphere, the left side of the body—it is said that left-handedness arises because the speech center, usually located in the left major hemisphere in right-handed individuals, is, in left-handed individuals, located in the right minor hemisphere. There are several serious objections to this claim. One is that about 2 percent of left-handers nevertheless have their speech center in the right cerebral hemisphere; and that about 2 percent of individuals who have their speech center in the right cerebral hemisphere are, nevertheless, right-handed.

More trenchant still is the fact that the many hundreds of right-handed children (and a few adults also) who have their entire, dominant, left cerebral hemisphere surgically removed because of tumor growth or irreversible brain damage do not become left-handed, nor indeed do they lose the power of speech.[28] (Least of all do they suddenly produce mirror writing!) The fact of the matter, which these operations make clear, is that *both* hemispheres are *both-handed*. Or, stating the position still more broadly, both cerebral hemispheres are always capable of all intellectual, spatial, and body functions. The (always provisional) location of specific functions in one or other hemisphere in the intact individual is really simply a matter of "administrative convenience"—the most rational use of the office space available, so to speak. There are no secrets between the hemispheres. All information generated is available, continuously and instantly, to either hemisphere.

Attaching the label of "handicap" to left-handedness is a more serious matter. There is, indeed, some justification for the use of the label in some cases. But this half-truth is allowed—or rather encouraged—to mask the full position.

First, it is quite clear that a higher incidence of left-handedness is found among the physically handicapped and the mentally retarded than among the general population. This increased incidence is only a matter of a few percent—a maximum of about 5 percent—but it is there. The reason is traceable to actual brain and nervous system damage. To put the picture at its crudest, if a person is paralyzed all down his or her right side, then he or she is necessarily left-handed. In less obvious cases, there is still some physical brain and nervous system damage—and the mind or psychology of the individual concerned salvages its best shot, as it were. In this work of salvage, of making the best use of the channels available, some would-be natural right-handers end up as left-handers.

Speaking of these damaged left-handers, Cyril Burt notes that they "show widespread difficulty in every form of finer muscular coordination . . . they squint, they stammer, they shuffle and shamble, they flounder about like seals out of water. Awkward in the house, and clumsy in their games, they are fumblers and bunglers at whatever they do. . . ."[29] Here, clearly, is the source of some of the bad reputation of the left. Will it do as an explanation of the material of this chapter? No, it will certainly not.

Like a very few other writers, I have long been occupied with the question of the gifted left-hander. Looking at any list of the famous, one is struck by the quite outstanding contributions of "lefties," academically, artistically, and in all branches of sport. In many cases they are the very byword of excellence, that is, they are *the* outstanding individual in their particular fields, as the following brief list of left-handers shows: Beethoven, Michelangelo, Leonardo da Vinci, Goethe, Nietzsche, Holbein, Chaplin, John McEnroe, Jimmy Connors, Pele, Babe Ruth. Those are some of the first-rankers—than whom there are no greater. Look even at the second rank: Cole Porter, Paul McCartney, Danny Kaye, Judy Garland, Betty Grable, Rex Harrison, Baden Powell, J. M. Barrie, Lewis Carroll, Rod Steiger, Olivia de Havilland, Landseer, Cicero—the list is virtually endless. Sandy in chapter 1 was left-handed, as we recall; and we shall also be meeting two other remarkable left-handers in chapter 19.

Clearly, these are not handicapped individuals. Nor are they gauche, awkward, maladroit. On the contrary, growing up in a world where every piece of equipment is designed for ease of use by right-handers—typewriters, scissors, telephones, doorknobs—as well as handwriting itself, and where the left is stigmatized as inferior, many of these disadvantaged lefties nevertheless easily out-achieve their environmentally-advantaged right-handed fellows.

This situation, and the need for an explanation of it, has not escaped everyone's attention—though it continues to escape that of modern Western psychology. Cyril Burt remarks in a puzzled way, "among bright and imaginative children of an emotional disposition, left-handedness is far from rare," but then he abandons the topic. (His use of the word "emotional" is, nevertheless, extremely interesting.)

This fact of the gifted left-hander has long been recognized, and sporadic references to it occur in ancient writings. One such reference in the Bible concerns a crack battalion of left-handed slingsmen who formed part of the army of the tribe of Benjamin. (Oddly enough, Benjamin means "the son of the right hand," so that there is a mystery within a mystery here. Later comments in this chapter throw some possible light upon it.) The text in question, Judges 20:16, states: "Among all this people there were seven hundred chosen men left-handed: every one could sling stones at a hair breadth and not miss." Nothing awkward or gauche about that lot, obviously. A further reference occurs in I Chronicles 12:1–2. Here a group is said to consist of "mighty men" (so again, nothing weak or womanish about them) who "could use both the right and the left in hurling stones and shooting arrows out of a bow, even of Saul's brethren of Benjamin." If the last phrase means "just like Saul's brethren of Benjamin," then we are dealing with a further group of skilled lefties (or ambidexters) from another tribe.

Were these ancient marksmen (and modern left-handed marksmen like Pele, Babe Ruth, McEnroe, and Connors) making use of the spatial abilities of the right minor cerebral hemisphere? Or were they rather employing the "left-handed" cerebellum, known to be involved in all fine movement and judgment of distance?

The question is posed again by some recent research findings concerning the handedness of American college students. Examining a total of 1045 students at an American college, J. Peterson established a 14.9 percent incidence of left-handedness among those majoring in music, a 12.2 percent incidence in the visual arts, and an incidence of only 4.4 percent among science majors.[30] Once again, is the explanation here simply that the arts involve the right minor cerebral hemisphere and the sciences the left major hemisphere?

Perhaps we might first usefully recall the close association between the arts and the unconscious noted in chapter 9, plus the strong sense of "daimon" experienced by artists. Jung has no hesitation at all in connecting the left, the unconscious, the emotions, and the feminine.[31]

As we have noted, however, fewer women than men are actually left-handed. A still more powerful argument against merely assigning the arts to the right minor cerebral hemisphere, however, is that there is no evidence whatsoever that the right hemisphere has any more connection with the unconscious or the emotions than the left major hemisphere—in other words, the minor hemisphere is not any more involved in dreaming, hypnosis, or meditation than the major hemisphere; and electrical stimulation of the minor hemisphere produces no autonomic reactions whatsoever, any more than does stimulation of the major hemisphere. The *cerebellum,* on the other hand, is very much concerned with the emotions and with the physical accompaniments of dreaming (see chapter 17). The cerebellum is, in fact, the headquarters of the autonomic (or self-governing) nervous system.

It *is* true that the left side of our face shows more emotion than the right.[32] But we can hardly assign that influence to the right *cerebral* hemisphere, since it has no special relation to emotion. We would have to think in terms, perhaps, of one of the *cerebellar* hemispheres.

Orthodox psychology and science have no explanation to offer of the phenomena we label as hypnosis, trance, possession and dreaming. There seems no chance that these can be accounted for by the interaction of the two cerebral hemispheres. But the idea of the "takeover" of the entire cerebrum by the cerebellum in the states mentioned has much to recommend it.

A further line of inquiry concerning left-handedness is ignored by modern western psychology. The incidence of left-handedness seems to differ sharply in different ethnic groups. In 1976 E. L. Teng and her associates examined a random sample of 4143 Chinese in Taiwan, made up of 1048 schoolboys, 1054 schoolgirls, 1025 male university students, and 1016 female university students.[33] The first two groups can be considered to represent the general population. The university system, however, is very highly selective, and the student groups represent the top 3 percent of the population in terms of IQ. Of the total sample population, 18 percent reported having experienced frequent requests to change hand use from left to right. As the authors emphasize, "only individuals who have a natural tendency for left-handedness . . . can be expected to experience social pressure for hand change." The conclusion is therefore that, allowed to follow their natural tendencies, 18 percent of Taiwanese would be left-handed. (Asiatics have much larger cerebella than Europeans, "very incompletely covered by the cerebrum."[34] Is this the explanation for the fact that among Chinese incidence of true left handedness is double that found in Britain and America?[35]) In current actuality, however, a scant 0.7 percent of the total population use the left hand for writing, and 1.5 percent use the left hand for eating. Nevertheless, the 18 percent of switched left-handers showed much use of the left hand for tasks other than writing or eating—which those who had reported no pressure for hand change (that is, the true right-handers) did *not* show. Conformity to the right-handed norm is only demanded in respect of the particular functions of writing and eating. In respect of other functions, where no social pressure is exerted, these 18 percent of individuals had retained their natural inclination to use the left hand in preference to the right.

There is much to be learned from these findings. First, they confirm indirectly the "commonly acknowledged" view of psychologists and anthropologists today that handedness is basically genetically, not environmentally, determined. Second, they are evidence of the injustice still done to left-handers (in all parts of the world). Third, they are evidence of an ancient and massively strong social tradition, for which we urgently need a coherent explanation.

One explanation of the world-wide fear and oppression of the left hand, and one that I have myself repeatedly suggested,[36] is the existence of an ancient, left-handed type of early man who was overrun and (partially) absorbed by the modern, right-handed type. (We could also argue that the earlier type had been very mystical.) The admixture of the two types might be different in different parts of the world, leading to different incidences of left-handedness. This view received support from some comments made as long ago as 1937 by Cyril Burt—he is quoting here not his own research but that of others.

> . . . it would appear that in prehistoric races, as in primitive tribes of today, the tendency to right-handedness was somewhat less universal than it is amongst ourselves. . . . An examination of throwing sticks yields proportions of 10 to 15 percent left-handedness, or slightly larger. Wm McDougall and others who have tested primitive communities . . . report a decidedly smaller preponderance of right-handed persons. The evidence from Paleolithic implements, cave-drawings and methods of working flints also suggests a high percentage of left-handers: one observer puts the proportion at least as high as 33 percent.[37]

That view of events is further tangentially supported by the existence of very old legends, which say that the left side was once good and lucky.

We ought to note, in conclusion, that the natural circling movement of left-handers is toward the left (anti-clockwise) and the natural circling movement of right-handers is toward the right (clockwise). Most interestingly, the Indian Tantrists call their worship of Shiva and Shakti the left-hand path, and the circling in occult groups (such as the whirling Dervishes) is also anti-clockwise—thus witches also dance "widdershins," and indeed to be seen dancing anti-clockwise around a church in medieval times was sufficient evidence for burning. This anti-clockwise movement is natural for a left-hander. Indeed, as we have seen at several points, reversals (of our standard normality) of all kinds are a feature of left-handedness. In *non*-automatic writing the left hand naturally prefers to write mirror writing (and from right to left across the page). Leonardo da Vinci and Lewis Carroll both produced such writing with ease, as do some of my own left-handed acquaintances. Finally, and very importantly, our own image in the mirror is left-handed (that is, if we are right-handed to start with) and it too produces mirror writing.

The left-handed creature from inner space who stares at us from the mirror is our other inner self. The vampire and the devil perhaps traditionally produce no reflection in a mirror because they *are* the reflection. It and they are probably, ultimately, the left-handed cerebellum.

─── 12 ───

A SHORT NOTE ON
UFOS

There are many strange and so far uncategorized events taking place in our skies.[1] While awaiting explanation, these serve as a vehicle for the longings and imaginings of the human unconscious mind—rather like heavenly Rorschach inkblots. However, the chances of the millions of reported sightings of unidentified flying objects having anything to do with visitors from outer space are effectively nil. They will remain so until and unless we have some fragment of manufactured extraterrestrial material for public inspection; or, even better, until some alien being walks openly amongst us.

It is very salutary to look back to the world-wide UFO epidemic of the 1890s.[2] This began in 1886 when the brazen notes of an "aerial trumpet" were heard by many in the neighborhood of lakes Ontario and Erie in Canada. Forty-eight hours later similar events were reported in Europe, and a week later in Asia. Observatories around the world cautiously admitted the possibility of an unusual electrical phenomenon. Less cautiously, an observatory in Finland reported the appearance at the center of the aurora borealis of a huge bird or aerial monster, from which showered corpuscles bursting like bombs. A Chinese observatory declared this phenomenon to be almost certainly a flying machine.

The detailed eyewitness reports from this era are particularly interesting. They emphasize how very thoroughly the alleged extraterrestrials were bound by humanity's then current conceptions of what was possible. By an amazing coincidence, the interstellar visitors (at any given point in history) have exactly reached the levels and types of expertise that we ourselves have evolved or can conceive of (in the 1930s UFOs took the form of airplanes). Thus the sighting reports from the 1890s speak of "a flying machine with a cigar-shaped fuselage and four metallic wings;" lights in the sky whose movement was suggestive of the "flapping of wings;" "a cigar shape with glass-enclosed gondola below;" "a combination of boat and balloon;" "a cigar-shaped four-winged object with a searchlight and fan-like 'wheels'"; "an airship with a pair of flapping wings"; and so on. Engine sounds were frequently heard, and sometimes machinery was glimpsed: "I could discern the wheels working." Voices (in America speaking English, and appropriate tongues elsewhere) were often heard, along with the sounds of singing. A farmer in Kansas reported that his cow was lassoed by a giant airship with "a great turbine wheel." From Chicago came a report of a UFO with wings and searchlight that tried to anchor atop City Hall.[3]

How pathetic and credulous these UFO reports sound today. About as pathetic and credulous as our own.

The psychological implications of the UFO phenomenon are of more interest. Many individuals who sight UFOs believe that these have come among us not by chance but with a clear purpose and intention. A significant proportion of sighters (usually called "contactees") believe that they personally have received messages from the UFO occupants to pass on to governments and humanity at large.

These messages are in the form of warnings. We, humanity, have begun tinkering with nuclear forces and with space travel. We have become very dangerous to the intergalactic community. We are about to contaminate the universe, both with radioactivity and with our insane appetite for warmongering and destruction. We are endangering the fabric of space–time, the future of the galaxy, or whatever. We must stop now, or be stopped. (Of course, in reality, if our sun and the nine planets all exploded together the rest of the universe would scarcely notice.)

A typical contactee case, chosen at random, is that of Frances Swan, an American and a devout seeker after philosophical truth. A strange, unidentified man came up to her one day in the local community hall on All Saints Day (Halloween) and spoke to her. He said that he had come specially to speak to her, and somehow he made a profound impression on her without saying very much. Six months later she began to hear in her left ear (the choice of the left is perhaps interesting) a shrill whistle, something like an A flat in tone. On 30 April 1954, she felt impelled to do some automatic writing. She wrote her first message: "We come will help keep peace . . . do not be frightened." Then in May: "We are on moon we are being watched constantly." The communicant or entity was Affa, from Uranus, cruising over earth in a spaceship 753,454 feet across. The mission of the ship was "to place a network of magnetic lines over the danger spots that will reinforce the wasted magnetism brought about by the sin and greedy hearts of men on your planet." Affa told Frances "not to be frightened at anything we may ask of you." She had been "selected to contact her people."[4]

This sample case, like the one that follows, suggests very much that what we have here is really the standard material of the séance room—the good intentions and the stern warnings of the "spirit guides" served up in long, candyfloss rigmaroles—but now with a topdressing of pseudo-science to make the situation more acceptable in, and appropriate to, our scientific age. (This currently widespread practice of adding the modern ingredient of pseudo-science to the old revelation pudding is one that the late Chris Evans and myself explored briefly in our pamphlet "Science Fiction as Religion."[5])

One UFO case that has received a great deal of publicity involves the alleged psychic Uri Geller and his amanuensis, Dr. Andrija Puharich. The details are given in Puharich's book *Uri*,[6] and their substance is briefly as follows. Uri Geller, as a child, was visited in his garden by a "huge, silent bowl-shaped object." A giant figure, apparently in a cape, suddenly stood between him and the bowl. A blinding ray of light came from this figure's head, and struck Uri so forcibly that he fell over unconscious. He so remained for several hours.

The implication is that this extraterrestrial visit endowed Uri with his alleged powers to bend metal paranormally, to read other people's thoughts, and so on. Years later Uri meets up with Andrija Puharich, a professional physiologist. Now the two of them are contacted by Spectra, the leader of "a Collegium of voices" who have traveled back in time from thousands of years in the future to help in the development of mankind—or not, as the case may be. For it seems that mankind is presently on trial: it is make-or-break time. The Spectrans fear that mankind "is an anxious and unacceptable race." The messages of the Spectrans, which materialize and dematerialize paranormally on tape, are full of pseudo-scientific jargon—but no *actual* science, as usual—and vague, generalized philosophy. The religious element is also clear: Uri and Puharich are constantly advised to pray.

In all the material offered (here and in other communications from various flying saucers and extraterrestrial speakers) there is no scrap of evidence that would make one consider the events narrated to be anything other than hallucinatory—if, that is, they are not outright lies. In either case, there is nothing in the UFO phenomenon that we have not already adequately dealt with under the heading of mediumship.

So much then for creatures from outer space: there really aren't any. But creatures from inner space, as we have seen, are a very different matter.

PART THREE

INTENTIONS

——— 13 ———
THE DYNAMIC
UNCONSCIOUS

I do not know what knowledge any of you may already have of psychoanalysis, either from reading or hearsay. . . .

Psychoanalysis maintains that there are such things as unconscious thinking and unconscious wishing . . . and incurs the suspicion of being a fantastic cult occupied with dark and unfathomable mysteries. . . . Nor can you guess yet what evolutionary process could have led to the denial of the unconscious, if it does indeed exist, nor what advantage could have been achieved by this denial . . . nor whether mental life is to be regarded as co-extensive with consciousness or whether it may be said to stretch beyond this limit. . . .

I shall positively advise you against coming to hear me a second time.

SIGMUND FREUD,
INTRODUCTORY LECTURES ON PSYCHOANALYSIS

Freud based his initial presentation to the general public of psychoanalysis and the dynamic unconscious, the *Introductory Lectures*,[1] on the most "flimsy" evidence he had—on what is now known as the "Freudian slip" or motivated error. For Freud well realized that once he could show in our own everyday lives any sort of purposive mechanism, any kind of intentional, organized activity in the mind, however slight, *other than that of normal waking consciousness,* the case for the unconscious mind was proven.

Freud was right in this approach. The publication of his first book *The Interpretation of Dreams*[2] in 1900 had been greeted with almost total indifference. The book sold less than four hundred copies in its first six years. But within another four years the medical, psychological, and scientific worlds were plunged into a controversy over psychoanalysis only equaled by the public storm over Darwin's *Origin of Species.* Today, while the narrower formulations of strict psychoanalytic theory (such as the Oedipus complex) are still under attack from academic psychologists (such as H. J. Eysenck), the basic tenets on which psychoanalysis is founded—the mechanisms of repression, denial, projection, rationalization, defense, regression, and so on—are part of those same psychologists' standard professional equipment.

The present book, in attempting to take the concept of the dynamic unconscious further than anything envisaged either by Freud or by modern psychology, also uses as a starting point the Freudian slip.

What the Freudian motivated error in its purest form shows is an intention or attitude on our part that is quite other than the intention or attitude in the matter in question that we express consciously, the attitude that we firmly and for the moment unshakably believe to represent our real opinion. In the Freudian error, then, are the first signs of an "alternative organization" and ultimately of an "alternative consciousness."

Examples of such errors serve better than any description of them, and the true state of affairs they reveal (in other people!) is very clear to all of us. So we have the wife who said: "My husband is much better. The doctor says he can now eat whatever I choose" (instead of "he chooses"); the lecturer who said, "Those who truly understand this matter can be counted on one finger—er—that is, on the fingers of one hand (the "one finger" being himself of course); the editor obliged to publish an article about a military man whom he disliked—the article carried the phrase "this battle-scared veteran," while the correction, with apologies, the next day stated "this bottle-scarred veteran;" the (as we realize) nervous messenger boy who knocked at the bishop's door, and responded to the bishop's "Who is it?" with "The Lord, my boy."

These are certainly amusing, perhaps trivial examples. It ceases to be a matter of amusement, however, when, for example, we miscall a lover's name, or, far worse, when the lover miscalls ours. Serious too are "forgotten" appointments, birthdays, and so on. The overlooked person quite fails to appreciate the "triviality" of the error. It is similarly no light matter when we lose, or break, something a lover or friend or relative has given us. The more significant or intimate the article—a wedding ring, perhaps—then so much the worse.

The seriousness, and more importantly, the motivatedness of the underlying situation is further emphasized when the "mistake" is repeated on more than one occasion (as we saw already with the editor above). So one married couple is invited by another married couple to dinner. The first couple forgets the engagement and goes to the theatre, leaving the second couple with an elaborately prepared meal and no guests. The first couple is abysmally apologetic: in compensation they invite the second couple to dinner with them at a later date. The second couple arrives to find an empty house. The first couple has gone out to the cinema. The same perseverance of the error is effectively seen when we write a date, an address, or whatever on a piece of paper (so as not to forget) and then lose the paper; or when we write an engagement in a diary but on the wrong day; or send an unsigned check as a present (having remembered, with some effort, the fact of the birthday itself).

Perhaps the most harrowing incident involving a Freudian slip, which will remove any still remaining smiles, is that of the Jewish man in prewar Germany, living as a non-Jew, who was entertaining a prominent Nazi for dinner. The man became fearful that his two sons were about to give away the secret of their Jewishness: so he said to them not, "Go into the garden, boys [*Jungen*]" but "Go into the garden, Jews [*Juden*]."

A sad rather than tragic example, which still stops short however of outright neurotic behavior, is Freud's story of the man who completely forgot his wedding day; and wisely, says Freud, decided to stay a bachelor for the rest of his life. In respect of this particular instance Freud writes:

> Everyone of us who can look back over a fairly long experience of life would probably say that he might have spared himself many disappointments and painful surprises, if he had had the courage to interpret as omens the little mistakes which he noticed in his intercourse with others, and to regard them as signs of tendencies still in the background.[3]

Freud takes us progressively from such everyday examples,[4] where the diehard skeptic can still protest that these errors are not important— or, at any rate, do not indicate any more extensive though still unconscious mental problem—to instances where we are dealing with serious disturbance and eventually with outright neurosis. There is no break in the continuum, however—only a steady increase in the implications involved, a growing realization of the latent complexities, of the *alternative organization of personality*, which must underlie the slip.

So he tells of a young married couple, how he heard the young wife laughingly describe her experience, that on the day after the return from the honeymoon she had been out for a walk with her sister, and had noticed a man on the other side of the street. "Look, there goes Mr. K," she remarked. She had forgotten that she had been married to this man for several weeks. The marriage, in fact, came to a very unhappy end some years later.

In their mildest form, the so-called "defense mechanisms" proposed and widely instanced by psychoanalysis—repression, denial, projection, and so on—resemble collections or aggregates of slips and misperceptions organized along particular lines and around a particular center, which persist over time. This at least is the appearance they present to an observer. These aggregates of slips and confusions are some of the outward signs of what is usually termed the unconscious (or neurotic) complex. Inwardly, what is said to have occurred at the unconscious level is that a cluster of consciously excluded or repressed contents have set up in business as a mini (or not so mini) opposition party to normal consciousness. (The rest of the unconscious mind need not be involved, however, and may be functioning normally.) The longer and more deeply excluded such repressed contents are, the more power they seem to gather, and the more they seem able to impose their own authority on conscious behavior—either in secret, guerrilla fashion, or finally in open, flagrant defiance of strong conscious attempts to ignore or control them.

The purpose of the present book is not to describe or define in further detail these and other well-established matters, which can be read of in any introductory text on psychology or psychiatry. For the purposes of the present book we want only to emphasize that the *principle* of organized, self-governing clusters of impulses outside, and in many ways independent of, normal consciousness is very well established—absolutely apart from and distinct from and prior to any context of the occult or the paranormal. Given that the notion (and of course, the fact of) unconscious impulse clusters exists, however, we are then entirely justified in using this concept as a possible basis for explaining self-governing paranormal "entities."

A brief word only, then, on one or two of the widely recognized defense mechanisms. The defense mechanism of projection, for example, involves seeing in the world around one that which is in reality only in oneself. Here, of course, is a possible explanation of visions, but we are speaking not so much of visual hallucinations, but of ideas.

In an experimental investigation each member of a group of students was asked to rate himself/herself and all other students, on a structured scale, in respect of meanness with money. All students identified one particular student as being especially mean with money. That student, however, rated himself as exceptionally generous with money, and everybody else as extremely mean. The actual meanness of this particular student (objectively obvious to all who knew him) was not perceived by him as being in himself at all, but as being in the world at large. However, such a fiction is not at all easy for the sufferer to maintain—since objective reality is constantly threatening to disprove it. He must, therefore, literally not notice others' acts of generosity—and, equally, must justify or rationalize his own persistent lack of it. He is, as a result, constantly quarrelling with others, is a social isolate, always under emotional stress, and so on. His behavior is to a greater or lesser degree neurotic, and will remain so until and unless the unconscious reasons for his meanness—probably connected with his early family life—are identified by a psychotherapist and gradually brought to his conscious awareness.

We can (and on the basis of many case studies do) assume that the student concerned was repressing the memory of very painful past experiences as a youngster—possibly of a marked lack of affection from one or both parents, or of too much love given by them to another child. The technical term "repressed" means the deliberate exclusion from consciousness of painful or repugnant or otherwise unwanted events. These are not genuinely forgotten, however. They persist at the unconscious level, distorting perceptions and threatening always to sabotage the individual's conscious control, perhaps even the total structure of his conscious personality. Similarly, we saw in chapter 7 how under hypnosis physical pain totally excluded from consciousness at the command of the hypnotist nevertheless persists unconsciously. For when the hand of the hypnotized person is allowed to write automatically, it protests about the pain that the unconscious mind is still experiencing. Neurotic individuals appear to be "dealing with" emotional pain and other difficulties in a similar way. However, repression does not in fact solve anything. It simply makes matters worse in the long run.

The unconscious mind, then, is a reality. It also has considerable powers of self-government and decision. It frequently overrides, contradicts or more subtly circumvents the wishes and orders of normal consciousness. (By the same token, however, the conscious mind also has powers and is also sometimes able to override and contradict the wishes of the unconscious—at the very simplest level, for instance, when we retain hold of a cup that is burning us badly in order not to damage a carpet. If the conscious mind were totally helpless there would be no conflict, nor indeed any possibility of conflict, between the two minds.)

The very relevant question for the present book is under what precise conditions is the unconscious mind able to override conscious intentions—neurosis is certainly one possible set of circumstances—and in advanced cases to become in fact the total opponent of all that the conscious mind wishes and stands for? Are there other circumstances? In this general context we should bear in mind that the name "Satan" means "an adversary, one who plots against another."

A common cause of the (neurotic) splitting away of the unconscious, or parts of it, from the conscious mind is that of denied or repressed sexuality, as many case studies testify. Such repression often occurs in narrowly religious homes, though not exclusively so. Victorian Britain, with its extremely black record of sexual repression in the fashioning of "good" men and women, was rife with the more extreme manifestations of neurosis and hysteria (see below). To Freud himself, living as he did in the Austrian equivalent of Victorian England, all neurosis was due in the final resort to repressed sexuality of one sort or another—the repressed desire of having the parent of the opposite sex as a sexual partner being said to be especially important. Freud really took no account of the possibility of repressed aggression, or repressed anything else, as a neurotic reagent—and indeed, in the Austria and Europe of his day aggression was not generally repressed in the psychoanalytic sense, even if some sought to control or channel it. (Karen Horney[5] and others later went on to suggest that any major *conflict of mental contents* could lead to repression and neurosis—for example, when a child is forced to choose between parents, or an adult to choose between marriage or career.)

In particular, however, neither Freud nor anyone else later sought to suggest *the repression of paranormal abilities* as a causal basis for neurosis—that is, for the splitting away from consciousness, and the consequent gathering to themselves of disproportionate separate powers, of aspects of the unconscious mind—a proposal that the present book makes herewith.

Already Freud himself—as a person, that is, not as a theorist—gives some support for the view just expressed. It is clear, firstly, that he had by no means fully come to terms with his own unconscious problems. He often fainted, for example, when his authority was challenged, or when differences occurred between him and those he regarded as father figures.[6] In a patient, of course, Freud would immediately have recognized such behavior as dissociative (see below). Did Freud therefore have problems in respect of his own aggression? Certainly he nursed a deep fear of the occult—"the black tide of mud of occultism," as he called it. Once again, had a patient of Freud's used such deeply emotive language on a subject Freud would immediately have become suspicious—but, apparently, his own unconscious blocks prevented him from detecting these warning signs in his own utterances. Was Freud, perhaps, a "repressed psychic?" The precise context in which Freud used his emotive phrase is in any case extremely interesting. Jung had been discussing religion and art with him, and had stated that aspects of these did not seem to him, Jung, to be reducible to repressed or sublimated sexuality, or to sexuality of any kind. This remark deeply distressed Freud so that he said:

> "My dear Jung, promise me never to abandon the sexual theory. That is the most essential thing of all. You see, we must make a dogma of it, an unshakable bulwark." He said that to me [Jung] with great emotion. . . . In some astonishment I asked him, "A bulwark—against what?" To which he replied, "Against the black tide of mud"—and here he hesitated for a moment, then added— "of occultism."[7]

Hesitation, in an appropriate context, is itself often an indicator of unconscious conflict and resistance.

There is, too, the famous account of the two poltergeist bangs in Freud's study when he and Jung were talking together. Jung had specifically asked Freud for his views on precognition and parapsychology in general. Freud then launched into a vehement rejection of these matters, in the shallowest of terms. Jung, angered by this unjustified snub, bit back a strong retort. However, Jung says that he now experienced a curious sensation, as if his diaphragm was made of iron and was glowing red-hot. There was then a loud bang from the bookcase, so loud as to frighten both men. Jung remarked that that was an example of the phenomena he had been referring to, and added that there would now be another bang. Sure enough, as he said the words, the second bang went off in the bookcase. Freud was very shaken. Perhaps Freud himself was the "medium" for that occult phenomena, or perhaps it was Jung; or possibly it was the two of them reacting together.[8]

Nevertheless, despite his general antipathy to the occult, Freud did come to believe in the existence of telepathy, and according to the biographer Frank Sulloway was only talked out of announcing his public support for the phenomenon by Ernest Jones, who argued that psychoanalysis already had enough hostility to contend with without that.[9]

Putting Freud entirely aside, however, the proposal is made here that the repression of paranormal powers may lead to a significant splitting of the unconscious from consciousness. It is, of course, not easy to untangle such alleged repression from any generalized sexual repression, but then, it is not easy to disentangle repressed sexuality and repressed aggression either, all these matters tending to be intricately tangled up together. However, if we imagine two parents, not necessarily religious, though they could be, who take a fairly cheerful view of human sexuality and "old Adam," and who do not object to an individual being outspoken and active (aggressive) in his own defense or a good cause, then we would not expect any child of theirs to be notably repressed in respect either of sex or aggression. But suppose a not particularly libidinous or aggressive child of theirs were genuinely fey—given perhaps to precognitive utterances or dreams, or to falling into dissociative states and trances, even to producing paranormal sounds or movements of objects—might the anxieties of these otherwise liberal parents be aroused? Might they not see this behavior as inadvisable, even devilish or mentally unbalanced? A strong anxiety reaction on their part would (as we know from many case histories) be quite sufficient to cause the child to reject and repress his or her, in this specific instance, emergent paranormality. Some of the individuals we are considering in this book, such as Mrs. W. D., or even Martyn Pryer, could perhaps be seen as examples of this kind of situation.

To revert to the main purpose of this chapter—we do, from psychology and psychiatry, have quite clear and indeed unassailable evidence, both in the case of normal and of outrightly neurotic individuals, (a) that the human unconscious mind does exist, (b) that it is *dynamic*—that it grows, changes, suffers tensions, adjusts or warps, is, in short, an organic, living system, and (c) that it has sometimes considerable—even very considerable—autonomy in the face of opposition from, or would-be control by, the conscious mind. The unconscious mind can, partly or (almost) wholly, temporarily or (almost) permanently, split away from the mind of normal consciousness to become a "mind within a mind" or an "organism within an organism." We have then coherent (or deliberately incoherent), systematized, continuous and extensive behaviors that are in no way desired, let alone commanded, by waking consciousness. Still more dramatic evidence of these will be presented in the next two chapters.

SPECIFIC NEUROSES

All neurotic behavior, as already suggested, is characterized by its defensive intent—that is, to defend some part of the personality against attack or hurt—but equally by the self-defeating consequences of its "solution." The "solution" is in fact the illness. Thus in agoraphobia the person concerned is afraid of going outdoors. The "solution" is to stay indoors. But this solution only means continuing to suffer from the illness permanently! The true solution involves, or would involve, finding out in psychotherapy what the outside world really represents to the sufferer at the unconscious level.

As part of their attempt to understand and treat neuroses, psychiatrists resort to systems of classification. As in the case of psychoses, however (see chapter 15), neurotic patients rarely oblige their physicians by presenting one neat set of symptoms, or by remaining permanently in any category to which diagnosis initially assigns them. Nevertheless, there are foci or contents in the personality, and in the history of the individual personality, around which symptoms tend to cluster; and an examination of case histories and presented symptoms does yield patterns of semi-reliable themes and influences. With caution, then, we can speak of types of neurosis.

The following classifications of neurotic disorder are commonly agreed: anxiety; hysterical (conversion and dissociative); phobic; obsessive-compulsive; depressive; depersonalization; hypochondriacal; other. Many of these terms are self explanatory. We can, however, be less rigid in our classifications by speaking instead of anxiety reactions (sudden, severe attacks of panic, apparently over nothing at all, or diffuse, generalized anxiety leading to stress illnesses like ulcers, palpitations, headaches), phobic reactions (as in agoraphobia and claustrophobia), depressive reactions, obsessive reactions (continually having to check that the taps are turned off, or the toilet flushed, or avoiding cracks in the pavements, and so on), fatigue reactions (always feeling tired without real cause), traumatic reactions (after a very bad car crash, for instance), conversion reactions (see below), hypochondriacal reactions (believing that one is continually suffering from a variety of illnesses not organically present), and so on.

Our interest in the present book centers chiefly on hysterical neurosis, both the conversion and dissociative varieties. (Though we recall, for instance, that Sandy had a *traumatic* car accident as a baby.)

The neurotic conversion of mental problems into other mental problems, which we come to shortly, is less common than the conversion of mental problems into motor and sensory ones. Thus in repressive societies "hysterical paralysis" is extremely common. Here a limb or an organ—commonly a hand or a leg—is paralyzed, and becomes completely unusable by the patient. There is, however, nothing organically or physically wrong with the limb, the problem is only functional. Nevertheless, this does not mean that the problem is not real. The sufferer *cannot* use the limb normally. It is exactly as if the limb were really organically damaged. Or, instead of paralyzed, the limb or area may be completely numb and without feeling (and it will be recalled that the inquisitors of medieval times searched for just such areas in those accused of witchcraft)—the sex organs, perhaps, or whatever. The sufferer has here *dissociated* himself or herself from the offending organ. It is no longer a part of the person concerned; he or she is no longer responsible for it or its nature. Conversely, however, an area of the body may become extremely painful to the touch. A similarly "additive" form of hysteria is hysterical pregnancy. A woman with this condition experiences all the physical and chemical concomitants of pregnancy (the swelling stomach, the cessation of periods, the morning sickness, and so on)—but there is no baby in the womb; it is empty. Additive symptoms are also seen in the person who has a permanently blushing face or a permanently erect penis. Some hysterical sufferers break out in a skin rash or boils whenever (say) they have to visit their mothers, or have asthma attacks when they approach the district where they grew up. Here we can recall the woman whose hip bled every time she saw her handicapped son put on his hip support. A mental problem can in fact be converted into virtually any form of physical symptom or illness—and so can be a very serious position indeed. The word "hysteria," incidentally, is from the Greek *hysterium,* meaning a uterus. The derivation is not an example of pure male chauvinism, for women do in fact suffer more than men from all forms of neurosis.

The amazing phenomenon known as multiple personality is a form (a very rare one) of conversion hysteria. Here very deep seated, extensive, and for the moment quite intractable mental problems are converted or dissociated into—another person! The "solution" is: "*I* don't have these depraved desires or these dirty sexual problems—*she* (or he) has them. It's all *her* (or him). I'm not like that at all." Within the one human brain, the nervous system or the mind constructs one or more additional, coherent, functional personalities who periodically take over consciousness and the entire body, and act out unacknowledged and unwanted desires and thoughts. The integrity, depth, and *differentness* of these fully functional usurping personalities is utterly staggering—and the whole of the next chapter is devoted to them. They necessarily call into question all currently accepted views on the structure of the human psyche.

Apart from the special case of multiple personality, we can already observe close parallels between the physical symptoms of conversion–dissociation hysteria and (a) the stigmata of the devoutly religious individual (chapter 8); (b) the production of wounds and rashes on the body under hypnosis (chapter 7); (c) the re-creation of childhood and other past body injuries in trance and psychotherapy (again chapter 7); (d) the bites and pricks on the body caused by poltergeists—including the "writing" on the face of the Sauchie child (chapter 3); and (e) the scars and marks on the bodies of Stevenson's "reincarnated" children and other reincarnation subjects (chapter 6).

Is it not a reasonable assumption that a similar psychological–physiological mechanism underlies all these various cases, even though there are differences between them at a more superficial level? It is now in fact proposed very firmly that the same mechanisms do, in principle, underlie all these perhaps at first sight distinct phenomena: that they all *are,* effectively, *one and the same phenomenon.*

SEX AND NEUROSIS

Sexual activity (like religious activity) has been a constant visitor to these pages—indeed the book started out with it.

A related and equally important matter concerns the relationship of sexual gender (i.e. maleness and femaleness) to (i) neurosis and psychosis, and (ii) the production of certain kinds of phenomena.

In respect of (ii) we have seen in chapter 9 a strong tendency for females to be associated with mediumship, and in chapter 3 a tendency, probably a significant tendency, for females to be associated with poltergeist phenomena. The latter tended to be females around the age of puberty (although one or two females around menopause were noted). There seems, however, little or no evidence for an association between the days of menstruation and poltergeist phenomena—though a censorship or nonreporting factor may be operating here. For from a wide variety of sources we have conclusive evidence of disturbed psychological and social behavior in the menstruating female, plus some evidence of increased vividness of dreaming and artistic creativity at that time.[10]

We are more immediately concerned here with the relation of maleness and femaleness both to neurosis and psychosis (considered in detail in chapter 15).

There is clear evidence that more females than males suffer from neurosis, and that more males than females suffer from psychosis. Two studies in America examined the psychiatric populations of (a) a rural county[11] and (b) a large urban district.[12] The first study reported the neurotics to comprise 60 percent females and 40 percent males, and the psychotics to comprise 57 percent males and 43 percent females. The second study returned similar figures in respect of the urban district. Such studies are regrettably few in number.[13] A. R. G. Owen however, unfortunately without giving his precise source, reports a further assessment of female neurotics outnumbering male neurotics by two to one.[14]

Fortunately these existing direct studies are supported by statistical analyses using the Minnesota Multiphasic Personality Inventory. The MMPI, as it is known for short, is a major personality test that has been very widely used and analyzed over a considerable period. Its structure and functions, strengths and weaknesses, are well understood. The test consists of a battery of questionnaires (or scales, as they are called). W. M. Wheeler and other analysts have established that the Hs, D, and Hy scales (representing hypochondriasis, depression, and hysteria respectively) are reliable for diagnosing neurosis; and that the Pa, Pt, and Sc scales (representing psychasthenia, masculinity–femininity of interest, and schizophrenia) are good for diagnosing psychosis. The three "psychosis" scales in turn correlate highly (and significantly higher than the neurotic scales) with the masculinity scale of the MMPI.

This observation that neurosis is commoner among women than men, and psychosis commoner among men than women, is an important item for the present book's general findings.

14

MULTIPLE
PERSONALITY

Cases of full multiple personality are rare. One recent reference entry speaks of "about a hundred"[1] authentic cases in the psychiatric literature, another of some two hundred.[2] These crucial cases, nevertheless, provide us with pivotal interpretations of much of the material of this book.

Multiple personality is a form of neurosis, specifically of hysterical neurosis. As already described in the previous chapter, in the hysterical individual mental problems are converted or dissociated into sensory and motor symptoms (paralysis, numbness, pain, wounds or whatever), or into other mental contents and behaviors (as in hysterical forgetting and amnesia). Often the converted-dissociated symptoms are rejected by the sufferer, that is they are not considered to have their source in his or her own body or personality; they have come in from outside like any normal illness. In fugue and amnesia states particularly, odd behavior is not just denied, but is totally forgotten.

It is important not to confuse extreme hysteria and the actually very different illnesses known as psychosis and schizophrenia (the subjects of the next chapter). Thus a hysteric, like a psychotic, may hear disembodied voices; but he or she *knows* that this is what they are, and is worried about them, realizing them not to be normal. (Of course, he or she will not agree that they represent some sexual problem, or whatever.) The psychotic, on the other hand, thinks it basically quite in order to hear such voices. (He is only worried, if at all, by the kinds of comments the voices are making.) Hence Carlotta in chapter 2 was initially diagnosed as hysteric, because she first agreed her visitations to be hallucinatory, but later as psychotic, when she began to consider her visitor to be real.

In the very extreme condition known as multiple personality, the neurotic problem takes the form not just of single, or even several, strange forms of behavior, but the form of a fully integrated alternative personality, sometimes even of several fully integrated alternative personalities. Such alternative personae will take over from normal consciousness for extended periods—sometimes for weeks or even months at a time, although sometimes just for an hour or two. During these periods the normal conscious personality disappears completely. It simply is not there. The later re-established normal personality has memory gaps in respect of events and the alternative time used up by the visitor. In particular, the sufferer will typically have no knowledge at all of the existence of the alternative personality.

It is very important to appreciate that what is being said here is not "a manner of speaking." The statements of the last few sentences are literally true. There is no playacting or pretense involved. The new take-over personalities have different beliefs, views, ideals, temperaments, ambitions, tastes, habits, experiences, and memories from those of the normal owner of the body in question, and from each other where more than one usurping persona is involved. The new personalities do not "merely" show different thoughts, views, and emotions; they exhibit different handwriting, can show different electroencephalograms (brain-wave patterns), and produce different performances on psychological projective, word-association, and vocabulary tests. Brain wave patterns, in particular, are impossible for anyone to fake.

Examples, as ever, are the best illustration.

In a well-known modern case, described in 1957 (though the actual events took place in the early 1950s) in the book *The Three Faces of*

Eve,[3] a woman, Eve White, was referred for psychiatric evaluation by her local physician. She had a difficult marriage. She was a devout Baptist, her husband a devout Catholic. Apart from the problems over the education of their child, Eve and Ralph White had an unsatisfactory sex life. Eve had begun to suffer from blinding headaches and occasional mental blackouts.

Her psychiatrists (Drs. Thigpen and Cleckley) describe the woman of the first several psychiatric sessions in great detail. She was gentle, even-voiced, almost withdrawn, with shoulders that stooped a little, and gave an impression of physical fragility. She was without humor, meek and humble—yet not actually spineless or lacking in conviction. Rather, her deep religious convictions made her the undemanding, unassertive, soul-searching, prayerful Christian.

Therapy over a year or so produced sometimes a lessening, sometimes a worsening, of the headaches. Her husband, however, now reported disturbed behaviors and mood swings on Eve's part. She had bought expensive clothes and completely forgotten she had purchased them, for example. She wrote a strange, disjointed letter to the psychiatrists, and in a subsequent interview admitted to hearing disembodied voices. She wept over this, realizing that she must be mentally ill.

At this point the first alternative personality, named Eve Black, abruptly emerged. The occurrence is described here in the doctors' own words.

The brooding look in her eyes became almost a stare. Eve seemed momentarily dazed. Suddenly her posture began to change. Her body slowly stiffened until she sat rigidly erect. An alien, inexplicable expression then came over her face. This was suddenly erased into utter blankness. The lines of her countenance seemed to shift in a barely visible, slow, rippling transformation. For a moment there was the impression of something arcane. Closing her eyes, she winced as she put her hands to her temples, pressed hard, and twisted them as if to combat sudden pain. A slight shudder passed over her entire body.

Then the hands lightly dropped. She relaxed easily into an attitude of comfort the physician had never before seen in this patient. A pair of blue eyes popped open. There was a quick reckless smile. In a bright unfamiliar voice that sparkled, the woman said, "Hi, there, Doc!"

With a soft and surprisingly intimate syllable of laughter, she crossed her legs, carelessly swirling her skirt in the process. She unhurriedly smoothed the hem down over her knees in a manner that was playful and somehow just a little provocative. From a corner of his preoccupied awareness the physician had vaguely noted for the first time how attractive those legs were. She settled a little more deeply into the cushions of the chair. The demure and constrained posture of Eve White had melted into buoyant repose. One little foot crossed over the other began a slow, small, rhythmic, rocking motion that seemed to express alert contentment as pervasively as the gentle wagging of a fox terrier's tail.[4]

We are principally concerned in the present book only with particular aspects of these manifestations. (Where before, for instance, have we found people speaking in unfamiliar voices? In connection, of course, with mediumistic trance in chapter 9 and hypnotic trance in chapter 7.) We shall not, therefore, pursue the story of Eve White and Eve Black in detail. However, several points in the Eve case must be emphasized.

One is that the now emerged Eve Black (as she was to be named) proved indeed to be the vibrant sex symbol her first manifestation suggested. Clearly (and without being simplistic about it) the persona and energy of Eve Black were composed in part of all the perfectly natural longings of the flesh that are every human being's birthright, but which the religious upbringing of Eve White (and her marriage to another equally religious individual) had denied—as well as the comparatively minor aspects of cheerful disrespect for cant and humbug, of having a good time for its own sake and just because you happen to be alive, that reasonable human beings know and accept. Thigpen and Cleckley in fact later describe Eve Black as a natural, fun-loving party girl.

An extremely interesting point for our own inquiry is that Eve White was very susceptible to hypnosis: she was a good subject. In one session Eve White was put into hypnotic trance, and Eve Black was then called by name and told to speak. The woman in front of the doctors opened her eyes and promptly "turned into" Eve Black—with her relaxed, buoyant posture, and brisk, husky voice. The doctors report that the subtle but complete change occurred in a moment, the body carrying out instantly and without trial or tentativeness its dozens of minute readjustments. This particular phenomenon we shall observe repeatedly in these cases. The first words Eve Black then spoke on this occasion recall for us, with a chill perhaps, the whole areas of demonology and satanism. She said: "Well, Doc, what you did just now sure made it easier for me to get out."

Later a third persona, Jane, emerged in the course of Eve's therapy, one quite unlike either of the other two personalities. Apart from the dramatic psychological differences, the authors note that Jane even somehow seemed to stand taller than the other two. Her walk and posture in any case were entirely her own. She had also a most impressive command of language, which far exceeded the abilities of the other two personae.

Turning to another famous case, that of Miss Christine Beauchamp, as reported by Dr. Morton Prince in his *Dissociation of a Personality* (first published in 1904; republished in 1978),[5] we find ample further confirmation of the links between multiple personality and the occult phenomena we have already considered.

Miss Beauchamp, as she initially presented herself for treatment, was as quiet, self-effacing, and reticent as Eve White, if not more so. (She "cannot be provoked into rudeness" and "bears in silence what others might resent.") She suffered from headaches, insomnia, bodily pains, and persistent fatigue and ate poorly. She presented, in all, four personalities. The first, BI, was known as Miss Beauchamp. BII was BI in the hypnotic state—substantially Miss Beauchamp herself, but without her reserve, lack of confidence, and neurasthenia. BIII was a personality known as Sally (and there are very interesting parallels between her and Eve Black). BIV did not have another name—although Sally called her "the Idiot." (It is not unusual for the dominant pseudo-personality to have some awareness of the other personalities, unlike the patient, who has none. In this respect, as in many others, the dominant pseudo-personality is much more effective and real than the patient.) Dr. Prince remarks that if he were not writing a serious psychological study he might be tempted to name the personalities as follows: BI—the Saint; BIV—the Woman; and BIII (Sally)—the Devil. Sally, however, as Prince emphasizes, is not to be understood as an evil being, merely a mischievous and immoral imp (much like Eve Black).

Prince further points out that each of the three major personae just listed had different health and constitutions—one more proof that we are dealing with something far more complex and radical than "mere imagination." BI had poor health; BIV was normally robust and capable of the usual physical exertions without ill effects; while BIII "is a stranger to ache or pain," she simply did not know what illness meant.

Morton Prince initially treated Miss Beauchamp by hypnosis. Like Eve, she proved a good subject. At first the therapeutic hypnotic sessions were fairly routine, but soon the other personae began manifesting in them. In no way, of course, did Prince suggest any of these personae to his patient.

The full course of Miss Beauchamp's tribulations and her therapy are not of direct interest to us. One single instance must satisfy us of the nightmare life that is lived by the person suffering from multiple personality. The normal Miss Beauchamp (BI) had a horror of spiders, snakes, and toads, loathing them with an emotion bordering on terror. One day she found in her room a neatly wrapped and tied box, which appeared to be a present. When she opened it six spiders ran out. She screamed and dropped the box, and the spiders scurried all over the room. It turned out that Sally had gone out into the country and gathered these spiders as a treat for Miss Beauchamp.

We move on now instead to an incident relatively late in the story that once more shows how literally the competing personae jockey for

position in the seat of consciousness and that links us with our more
general considerations throughout the book.

> BIV, in a depressed, despondent, rather angry frame of mind, was
> looking at herself in the mirror. She was combing her hair, and at
> the same time thinking deeply over the interview she had just had
> with me in regard to her ultimatum to Sally (BIII). Suddenly she saw,
> notwithstanding the seriousness of her thoughts, a curious, laugh-
> ing expression—a regular diabolical smile—come over her face. It
> was not her own expression, but one that she had never seen before.
> It seemed to her devilish, diabolical and uncanny, entirely out of
> keeping with her thoughts. (This expression I recognized from the
> description to be the peculiar smile of Sally, which I had often seen
> on the face of BI or BIV.) BIV had a feeling of horror come over
> her at what she saw. She seemed to recognize it as the expression
> of the thing that possessed her. She saw herself as another person
> in the mirror and was frightened by the extraordinary character of
> the expression.[6]

BIV, trying to keep her nerve, now hit upon the idea of speaking to
the creature in the mirror by using automatic writing (a very fashionable
activity at that time). Accordingly BIV obtained a pencil and paper and,
holding the pencil, asked the thing, "Who are you?" The reply that came
is of the greatest interest: "A spirit."

In a later session of automatic writing, in the presence of Morton
Prince, who was questioning BIV's *hand*—that is, was questioning Sally—
about various incidents, the hand wrote: "I am a spirit. You know it is
true" and "God will punish you for your levity." These clear links with
the standard product of the mediumistic session will be dramatically confirmed and amplified in a moment—but before that a concluding word
about Sally.

As has already been demonstrated, these alternative personalities
are incredibly real and three-dimensional. We have indeed no firm *a
priori* grounds for distinguishing them from a real person—especially,

perhaps, when some of them display different EEG patterns from the person they displace; and in fact we must strongly doubt that the Freudian psychoanalytic explanation of a "small part" of consciousness having been detached and repressed by the sufferer of the neurosis will do at all. We appear to have something far more on hand than that (and, of course, we are not a million miles from Carlotta's incubus). What the present book will in fact finally be proposing is the outgrowth of an extra consciousness, and extra person or persons, on the "stem" of the unconscious—as if a single-stemmed flower, having produced and developed its usual single bud, then begins to grow and develop new buds, which also open to become full flowers.

In any event, can we fail to be daunted by the letter that Sally (during one of her periods of full control) wrote to Dr. Prince, when, in therapy, it began to look as if Miss Beauchamp was going to be able finally to reassert herself: "Please forgive me again . . . and let me *stay. Please, please, please.*" [Sally's italics]

The reader can study the full reality of Sally and her delightful, immoral charm in Morton Prince's book—and reflect that a medieval society confronted by this phenomenon, as it often enough was, could only think in terms of discarnate demons and spirits. Indeed, can *we* do less—except to make the "slight" adjustment of realizing that these "spirits," these *new people* are not from outer space, not from somewhere beyond, but from the interstellar inner reaches of the human personality.

Sally, again, confirms this view—and again gives quite heartrending evidence of her realness. She hatched the idea that if she could only read French, and become well educated, she would not be looked down on as "nothing but a subliminal" and be allowed to stay. She repeated often that she had "just as much right to stay as they had."

We turn now to other aspects of the (real) Miss Beauchamp's behavior, long prior to her breakdown and submission to therapy. As a child Miss Beauchamp had frequently had visions of the Madonna and Christ. She herself believed that she had actually seen them, and that they were real. She used to pray whenever she was in trouble of any kind, and then would come a vision of Christ. It did not address her in words, but made signs and gazed at her lovingly and with understanding. Then, afterwards, whatever difficulty she was in would somehow solve itself. On one particular occasion she had lost a key. Her vision of Christ led her along the street and into a field where, under a tree, she now found the key. Apart from the visions themselves, Miss Beauchamp used as a child constantly to have the sense of a presence near to her—Christ, the Madonna, or a saint.

Then, during her therapy with Dr. Prince, the adult BI had an active vision of Christ in connection with a current problem. She had lost a check and had spent five days looking for it without avail. On that fifth night she awoke at 4 A.M. with the sense of a presence in the room. When she got out of bed she saw a vision of Christ. The vision, as before, did not speak, but smiled at her. Now all her anxiety over the check vanished. The figure led her over to the bureau. Here she at once found the check in the top drawer—wrapped inside some of her sewing.

Next day, under hypnosis, Dr. Prince questioned BII about the matter. BI had claimed to have put the check into a book. BII, however, said that BI had been standing with the check in one hand and a book in the other, with the full intention of inserting the check, when a knock had come at the door. The check and book were put down on a table and forgotten. Later BI had gathered up her sewing, inadvertently wrapping up the check inside it, and placed the whole bundle in the bureau drawer.

These incidents are full of instruction for us.

First, we have visions of Christ and the Madonna on the part of a devout little girl such as are usually acclaimed by religious adults as evidence of divine intervention, and even considered to be adequate grounds for the setting up of a holy shrine (as in the case of Lourdes in the mid-nineteenth-century, or more recently at Banneux, Belgium, in 1933 and at Trefontane in Italy in 1947).

But as it happens, this little girl as an adult has a severe neurotic breakdown. Then she has a further vision of Christ, who helps her to find a lost check. We can choose: (a) to regard the holy visions of Miss Beauchamp, and by inference all other holy visions, as mere hallucinations, simply products of the human mind or (b) to regard Miss Beauchamp's holy vision (and all such others) as real, while discounting the fact of Miss Beauchamp's later illness. We then still have to come to terms with the idea of a Christ who has time to help find checks. In Miss Beauchamp's case, our most reasonable interpretation is hallucination. Why should the case be different in other holy visions?

Second, as already shown in respect of hypnosis and the memory of "past lives," we again have clear evidence here that the unconscious mind sees and records everything in our lives, on its own account, and quite independently of consciousness. The conscious mind of Miss Beauchamp believed she had put the check in a book, taking firm intention for completed action, but the unconscious mind observed the check being picked up with the sewing.

Third, we see once more how frequently the phenomena discussed in this book tend to affect and involve the deeply religious. We reach a point, in fact, where we might with much justice argue that religious behavior itself must be a neurosis.

Fourth, the previous incident of Sally's face appearing in the mirror links us with every aspect of the material already discussed in respect of automatic writing.

The frequent use of the words "sudden" and "abrupt" in describing the occurrence of personality change in multiple personality is striking. Harking back for a moment to Eve, for example, Thigpen and Cleckley describe a typical incident: ". . . before the tentative voice of Eve White could make its first comment on the experience . . . Eve Black burst out suddenly and unbidden." The change itself also seems to the observer to reach right down into the basic biological mechanisms of personality.

The comment that follows concerns Billy Milligan, another famous and this time recent case.[7] Billy, the illegitimate son of a Catholic mother and a Jewish father, was persecuted by his later stepfather to drive out both Catholic and Jewish influences. Billy was perpetually thrashed and subjected to sexual abuse, including anal intercourse, by his new parent. As with still another well-known modern case, Sybil,[8] where the young girl in question was sexually tortured by her schizophrenic mother, Billy's story reads like an experimental attempt to induce fragmented personality. Yet a further instance of early traumatic sexual experience leading to multiple personality in adult life is reported by Ernest Hilgard.[9] The girl, Kathy, was raped, both anally and orally, by an elder brother, at the age of seven. Then, when she reached home after this frightening event, her father beat her for being late. At the age of ten Kathy saw her twelve-year-old sister raped by several boys, and at the age of seventeen was herself raped by three boys.

However, concerning the point of personality change in Billy, an observer notes:

> Those witnessing the moment of personality change find the process eerie and unforgettable. Milligan stops talking in mid-sentence and freezes. His eyelids flutter uncontrollably, his face smoothes out for an instant, turning strangely ageless.[10]

Such dramatic and fundamental change can be observed (a) in hypnotic subjects regressed to a "past life," (b) in mediums in deep trance, and (c) was observed, and photographed, in Carlotta. Such change must have been seen and noted in medieval and ancient historic times, and probably ever since man evolved, in those said to be possessed of demons and devils. Probably indeed the world-wide religious edifice of demons and angels has no other basis.

Drs. Boris Sidis and Simon Goodhart, writing originally in 1904, but republished in 1968,[11] have much further interesting material in this area. They tell of one patient, the Reverend Thomas Hanna (again the religious connection), who was able to sense and describe the two personalities within him fighting for possession of his consciousness. Subsequently he reported his inner experiences to Drs. Sidis and Goodhart, his therapists.

Q. How did the two [sets of] memories appear to you?

A. As two different persons.

Q. Which life did you prefer to accept?

A. I was willing to take either. The struggle was not so much to choose one as to forget the other. I was trying to find out which I might most easily forget. It seemed impossible to forget one; both tried to persist in consciousness. It seemed as if each memory was stronger than my will. . . . Just before lunch yesterday, in the psychological laboratory, I chose the secondary life; it was strong and fresh and able to persist. The primary was more clouded and easier to subdue. I tried alternately to throw each away, and succeeded at last in throwing away the primary and emerged into the secondary state. At Dr. G's office I had the same struggle over again . . . I wanted to be alone to decide which life to give up.[12]

In this account we see once more how very real the pseudo personality can be even when compared directly with the original personality (yet, in view of what we have seen here, how much value or permanence can we in fact assign to any "original" personality?). Mr. Hanna was finally unable to abandon either of the two personae, but succeeded in permanently uniting them, a very satisfactory outcome from the therapeutic point of view. One very interesting point in this case, as described, is that consciousness itself seems somehow to function independently of any personality whatsoever. This is an extremely interesting possibility, which has already been discussed in an earlier book[13] and to which we shall refer again.

Yet a word of warning, too, on the permanence of any personality synthesis. In the case of Eve, the third personality, Jane, had seemed able to subsume or accommodate both Eve White and Eve Black. Jane appeared from every point of view to be the *real* Eve (who had been fractured into White and Black, but was now made whole again, with a much enhanced personality). As the new Jane, Eve remarried and for several years lived a successful and integrated life. Then Jane wrote to her former university for a testimonial. Alas, she had never been at that university—only her cousin had. "Jane" was another—and quite marvelous, we must agree—false or perhaps "false" personality. One begins to want to start writing every word in double quotes for the apparently hard certainties of Western mainstream psychology and Western personality theory appear to be nothing of the kind.

Eve White (or whichever of her various names we prefer to use) then underwent a very severe breakdown, lasting some twenty years, and now told of in a new book.[14] Around twenty identifiable personalities came and went and switched on the stage of this unfortunate woman's mind, outdoing the sixteen or so personalities attributed to Sybil.[15] Truly, as the Biblical Gadarene madman said, our name appears to be legion.

15

PSYCHOSIS, SCHIZOPHRENIA, AND AUTISM

The very large majority of both psychologists and psychiatrists consider psychosis, of which schizophrenia is one special variety, to be radically different from neurosis. It is true that it is sometimes difficult to distinguish between an extreme neurosis, like multiple personality, and a psychosis, but such exceptional cases apart, the differences between these two major forms of mental illness remain both clear and persistent. In neurosis there is a difficulty with or an alienation from some aspect of life and society, but in psychosis there is a sharp, clear break from the objective reality that the rest of us (both normals and neurotics) perceive. The psychotic is not simply out of his mind. He is out of our world.

Various *bons mots* have been coined to bring out the basic difference involved. For example, it is said that neurotics build castles in the air, but psychotics live in them. Or a neurotic will say that he is not going to get up to go to work, because he hates the world and it hates him. But the psychotic will say that he does not have to get up because he has stopped the sun from moving.

When we hear the stories and complaints of psychotic individuals, the bizarreness, the impossibility, the sheer madness of their claims is immediately obvious to us. A woman says that her neighbors are using cosmic rays to torture her. Another says that the dentist has inserted a miniature radio into her teeth in order to spy on her. A man tells us that the Queen has given instructions for him to be secretly poisoned. Another that the bus conductress felt his arm this morning to see if he had been masturbating. Finally, most people suffering from psychosis seem not to know that there is anything wrong with them, no matter how unusual their behavior may be to others and in terms of objective reality. Neurotics, by contrast, do appear to know that something is wrong with them (though they may well reject other people's assessment of it) and want, in some sense, to be rid of their symptoms.

A major division within psychosis itself is between the organic psychoses and the functional psychoses. In organic psychosis actual physical brain or nervous system damage or deterioration is detectable, whereas in the functional psychoses (which include schizophrenia) it is not—or at any rate, not by any methods currently known to us.

Actual brain damage may be due to any of a wide range of factors—accidents, tumors, the process of growing old, alcoholism, drug-taking, and so on. These organic psychoses are of some interest to the present book, in that they frequently involve hallucinations—the perception of people or animals or creatures that are not physically there. However, the interest is diminished when we appreciate that organic psychosis also involves considerable general personality and mental deterioration and confusion, even delirium. There is a marked reduction in intelligence, understanding, memory, concentration, and attention. This general loss of mental faculties is, however, not one that we associate with mediumship in particular or psychic phenomena in general.

The functional psychoses, especially perhaps schizophrenia, are of much greater interest to us. These psychoses often involve highly intelligent individuals, including outstandingly creative people—Van Gogh, Strindberg, and Hölderlin are well-known instances.

One group of functional psychoses, the affective psychoses, has a strong emotional basis—manic depression, depressive psychosis, and mania (hypomania) being the three major forms, though some authorities feel that all types are simply forms of manic depression. As it happens, these affective (emotional) psychoses are commoner in women than in men, a statement that runs counter to the general statement in chapter 13 that psychosis in general is more common among men than women. The novelist Virginia Woolf was a gifted writer who finally succumbed to manic depression. Her husband, Leonard Woolf, wrote subsequently:

> ... then suddenly the headache, the sleeplessness, the racing thoughts would become intense and it might be several weeks before she could begin again to live a normal life. . . . There were moments or periods during her illness when she was what could be called "raving mad" and her thoughts and speech became completely uncoordinated. . . . During the depressive stage all her thoughts and emotions were the exact opposite of what they had been in the manic stage . . . she scarcely spoke, refused to eat, refused to believe she was ill. . . .[1]

(Virginia Woolf, after some earlier attempts at suicide, drowned herself in the River Ouse in 1941.)

Involutional melancholia (sometimes also involutional paranoia) resembles the depression end of manic depression (and, again, is three times commoner in women than men), except for its onset late in life. All these depressive psychoses cause a marked decrease in sexual desire. Sexuality, in this negative sense, is again implicated in involutional paranoia, a condition that attacks mainly unmarried men in their forties and fifties who have made a poor sexual adjustment. This is a logical system of delusions concerning plots and conspiracies that is well and reasonably argued (here is the difference from paranoid schizophrenia—see below) once the initially false premises are accepted.

In all psychoses, however, as in all neuroses, patients seldom exhibit a neat, textbook pattern of symptoms, and quite often shift out of one diagnostic category into another altogether. With that caveat, probably the most relevant form of described psychosis for the present book is schizophrenia.

SCHIZOPHRENIA

Schizophrenia is the most frequently made diagnosis among the major psychoses, involving some 20 to 25 percent of first admissions to mental hospitals. Its onset usually takes place before the age of forty—so therefore *could* in principle concern almost all our poltergeist subjects.

The word "schizophrenic," though it means "split mind," has no connection at all with the phenomenon of multiple personality that, to emphasize this once again, is a neurosis, and specifically a form of conversion hysteria (see chapters 13 and 14). The "split" in schizophrenia is between thought and feeling. In the schizophrenic, thought, behavior, and feelings have all come adrift from one another. There is a preoccupation or, more accurately, a continuous involvement with fantasy rather than reality. Schizophrenics "know their own unconscious." They may speak "word-salad"—a continuous flow of word association and puns, of references and allusions bouncing one off another like a display of fireworks, sometimes incoherent and completely unintelligible, at other times invested with flashes of mysteries and poetic insight, or half-insight, where the listener feels he is being witness to revelations. Indeed, the utterances of schizophrenics are sometimes published as poems or poetic prose. As Andrew Crowcroft remarks, "the boundaries between conscious and unconscious, between outside world and inner world are dissolved . . . [schizophrenics] are dreaming while awake."[2] The same features are observed also in another modality, when schizophrenics paint—the confusion and whirling of colors and images are very close to great art, and occasionally *are* such. We see this above all in the later paintings of Van Gogh. But sadly, when the disease worsens, the images of schizophrenic painting pass even beyond the elastic boundaries of art into chaos and incoherence.

The relevance of these matters to the increased creativity observed in hypnotic regression (chapter 6), in automatic writing (chapter 5), and in mediumship (chapter 9), especially to the "speaking in tongues" of mediums, mystics, and saints, has already been noted. Yet the medium, the mystic, and the hypnotized are not schizophrenic in any psychiatric sense.

In schizophrenia, there are said, clinically, to be four major divisions:

(a) simple schizophrenia, involving (hence the name) simple thinking patterns, shallow emotions, and a noticeably reduced level of
   general activity;

(b) hebephrenic schizophrenia, where condition (a) worsens into
   silly or bizarre behavior, delusional beliefs, hallucinations, and
   the hearing of voices not audible to others;

(c) catatonic schizophrenia, involving grotesque bodily posturing, in
   which the sufferer may become completely frozen, hence also the
   condition of mutism, extreme compliance, and loss of voluntary
   activity—punctuated, however, by impulsive episodes of exces-
   sive movement and excitement;

(d) paranoid schizophrenia, involving like (b) illogical, unreal hallucinatory thinking and bizarre delusions—of persecution, or of
   being a great personage like Napoleon—and, again, voices that
   no one else hears.

The voices and hallucinations of (b) and (d) do, at first sight, remind
us once more of the spiritualist medium and the psychic. These also hear
voices that others do not, and see spirits, ghostly visitors and so forth,
not usually visible to others. The basic differences between the schizophrenic and the medium will be apparent from the comments in chapter
18. Yet, at the same time, we must beware of absolute distinctions. As
J. Dominian remarks: "Among candidates offering themselves for the
religious vocation, there is invariably a percentage who, in the course
of time, will develop schizophrenia."[3] There is a percentage too, as we
know, who will develop multiple personality.

Autism is the name given to psychosis and schizophrenia in children. These illnesses in children are very like those of adults, though not
wholly identical, perhaps simply because we are dealing with a prepu-
bertal organism instead of a postpubertal one. The psychotic child, in
any case, has never passed through the normal, formative experiences
that even adult psychotics once knew.

Andrew Crowcroft describes the psychotic child as follows:

A psychotic child fails to relate emotionally in a proper fashion, or at all, to other people. He seems unaware of his own identity, sometimes repeatedly examining some part of his body, as though it did not belong to him. Such a child may only play with one object in a fixed way, a way perhaps quite odd. In some cases he seems to strive to keep everything around him—furniture, toys—exactly the same. Reactions to pain, or to things seen or heard, are sometimes abnormal. George, for example, could fall over quite hard and not cry.

There may be episodes of acute anxiety, difficult or impossible for his parents to understand. Speech may never be acquired, or may be lost. The general behavior of the child is unusual, his activity being greater or much less than in a normal child. He may exhibit bizarre postures, or show curious mannerisms and carry out repeated rituals of an apparently meaningless kind.[4]

More technically, an autistic child shows: (a) severe impairment of social relationships, (b) severe impairment of language, (c) evidence of rigidity and inflexibility of thought processes—evidenced in particular by ritualistic behavior, and (d) the early onset of symptoms, usually before the age of thirty months.

There is a famous case of childhood autism that is of great interest to the present book. It concerns a girl called Nadia. All the information and quotations that now follow are taken from Lorna Selfe's book, *Nadia: a Case of Extraordinary Drawing Ability in an Autistic Child.*[5]

Nadia's parents were Ukrainian immigrants, and she was born in Nottingham, England, in 1967. The pregnancy and birth were in themselves uneventful. Soon, however, her mother reported that she was "unlike other children." She was unresponsive to stimuli. She seemed also to have poor muscle tone, and would lean against people and objects, as if for support, when sat up. Her first words appeared at nine months, and she soon had a vocabulary of about ten words. But at eighteen months she not only had not acquired any further words, but was using her ten words less and less frequently. She did not walk until two years of age. She was inattentive, heedless of danger, and generally difficult to control.

Nadia came to Lorna Selfe's attention when she was six years old. She was large for her age (her bone age was in fact seven or eight years), clumsy, slow in her movements, and poorly coordinated. Social overtures to her were largely ignored, neither did she respond to commands and instructions. Such response as she would make would be merely to repeat what had been said (ecolalia), e.g., "Hello, Nadia." During the twice weekly two-hour sessions with the psychologist, either at home or school, over a five-month period, Nadia used only some ten words of vocabulary.

In her special school (which she started at four and a half years) she could "only eat with a spoon" . . . "was sometimes destructive and frequently had uncontrollable attacks of screaming" . . . "had regular temper tantrums when she would scream and shout uncontrollably for two or three hours at a time." However, "her typical behavior in the classroom was one of withdrawal into her own private world, with passive cooperation toward her teacher. She would sit for half an hour staring into space or wander slowly and aimlessly about the room."

The record of this time continues the sad, detailed picture of a severely damaged child. "She will not listen to stories . . . when disturbed or confused she will suddenly talk jargon to herself—no one can understand what she says." She "can dress herself" but "is liable to put her clothes on the wrong way round" and could "not manage large press-studs." She had "no fear of ordinary dangers, and cannot be trusted not to run into traffic or into a moving swing." And perhaps the saddest remark of all: "She can unwrap a chocolate bar without dropping the chocolate."

This is the child whose drawings we now discuss.

Nadia had begun drawing "suddenly" at the age of three and a half. Nadia, incidentally, is *left-handed*. From the very outset her mother was impressed with her daughter's dexterity and skill in art. Lorna Selfe writes:

Nadia used fine, quickly executed lines. Her motor control was highly developed, judged by her speed and the accuracy of execution together with a general deftness. She did not need to look at the line she had just drawn while surveying the movement of her hand at the same time—as is the case with many infants. Her lines were firm and executed without unintentional wavering. She could stop a line exactly where it met another despite the speed with which the line was drawn. She could change the direction of a line and draw lines at any angle towards and away from the body. She could draw a small but perfect circle in one movement and place a small dot at the centre.[6]

It was clear that Nadia well knew what she was doing and was fully aware of the effects she achieved. She would examine her drawings with obvious pleasure, moving her head to study angles, at the same time babbling with glee and shaking her hands and knees in delight. She would frequently be inspired by a picture in a book, rather than by life, although her pictures were not copied. She would often draw in the absence of the original inspiration and develop the theme in a series of pictures. Her favorite subjects were certain animals, notably horses (often with riders), and human figures, both sometimes caught in motion.

The drawings themselves are absolutely amazing and, of course, must be seen. Over a hundred of these, drawn between the ages of three and a half to eight years, make up the greater part of Lorna Selfe's large-format book. The skill of some of the horse drawings, seen head-on in movement, would "tax the skills of professional artists," and the studies of human figures sitting with crossed legs could come from any artist's notebook, perhaps even from Leonardo's.

Calculated solely on the basis of her drawings (for which standardized procedures exist), Nadia's IQ was 160. This figure is into the range of genius.

At the time Lorna Selfe's book was written Nadia was nine years old. Her language and social communication had improved, and she could handle simple numbers. She now seldom draws spontaneously, however. Occasionally she draws portraits of her classmates that succeed in capturing something of their likeness, not the easiest thing in the world to do, and still a remarkable talent. But one can no longer call Nadia's talent "unbelievable."

Nadia's drawing from some points of view does recall to us the "automatic" drawing of Matthew Manning, Luiz Gasperetto, and other mediums (chapter 5), the ability of Rosemary Brown to compose music in her dissociated state (chapter 9), as well as the unexpected talents in writing and music displayed by Anita Mühl's hospitalized psychotics (chapter 5). There are of course many differences between these various manifestations, but there are points of contact also.

Can we see, at any rate, that under slightly different conditions, Nadia's totally remarkable drawing abilities at the age of three-and-a-half—and which appeared "suddenly"—might have been considered as a case of the child's personality being taken over by a "discarnate spirit"? Indeed, had Nadia been a normal girl in other respects, she *herself* might have perceived her behavior as a takeover by (say) "an invisible playmate." Sometimes, while drawing, Nadia would fall into a staring reverie for several minutes. Such behavior could readily be interpreted as a "mediumistic trance," quite apart from Nadia's other oddnesses; her left-handedness alone could have pointed to a possibly occult motivation.

We are very fortunate in having the in itself unfortunate fact of Nadia's autism, plus the fact that she was observed by competent Western physicians and psychologists from the outset. There is really nowhere for either the "discarnate spirit" or the "reincarnation" hypothesis to creep in. Instead we have a most remarkable piece of behavior by the human nervous system, one that enables us to cast yet again strong doubt on spirit hypotheses in other cases. The possibility that Nadia's precocious artistic abilities in fact had their origin in that part of the brain we call the cerebellum will be considered in later chapters.

One final interesting parallel comes from Ian Wilson,[7] who notes that Nadia's loss of much of her ability, and her loss of interest in it, somewhat resembles the cessation of fantasies and the loss of interest in themselves as "reincarnated beings" of the young children studied by Ian Stevenson.[8]

16

THE NATURAL
HIST⊕RY ⊕F PSYCHICS

Despite an intense interest in spiritualism and paranormal phenomena throughout Europe and North America for well over
a hundred years, there exists not a scrap of information on the natural
history, or even the case history, of the psychic human being. There is, in
other words, no answer to the question: what kind of person develops
into a psychic?

There can be no substitute for a national or international survey of
existing psychics, such as the various Societies for Psychical Research
and the Spiritualist communities could readily undertake, but that they
show no signs whatsoever of undertaking. In this chapter, therefore, we
can do no more than give some indications of what such a survey might
reveal.

Some psychics emerge in the context of strongly religious families.
Others, however, like myself, appear from emphatically non-religious
backgrounds. Contrary also to popular (mainly religious) opinion, it
is not only the sexually abstinent (as in the case of saints) or sexually
underendowed persons who manifest psychic abilities. Some psychics
are intensely sexual, as we see in some of the instances to follow.

All the really obvious clues to psychic ability, however, appear to have been totally overlooked. For instance, it occurred to me many years ago that any sample of psychic individuals (such as mediums) would show a high incidence of left-handedness, both themselves and also among their immediate blood relations. (Why has this totally obvious idea not occurred to everybody in the field, given the role of the left and the left hand in the history of the occult?)

A relevant example involves my own family. I am not myself left-handed, but my brother was. In Canada I have a niece whom I lost touch with for many years. Recently she contacted me, and I asked her if any of her children were left-handed. She wrote:

Trisha, my eldest of three daughters, is left-handed. As a very young child she used to tell me of these pale clouds of grey mist that would follow her sometimes. No one could see them but her. I would sometimes see her running for something, and she would tell me it was the mist. Then later she would wake me at night and tell me that a man was sitting on her bed, but she did not know who he was. She was then six years old.

Apart from the link with left-handedness, this illustration (like others following, and Ruth's story in chapter 10) suggests that psychic abilities run in families, and are genetically, not environmentally, induced. The clouds of mist here further recall Ena Twigg's "misty people" (see p. 188), while the visiting figure strongly reminds us of Ruth's early history.

As the brief survey of this chapter bears out, the psychic individual shows from earliest childhood an intense involvement in, and usually love of, what we might term "spiritual" (but not necessarily religious) and imaginative matters, ranging from a love of nature and natural things, to that of the actual supernatural and fairy world (this often being accompanied by daylight visions of supernatural figures), as well as intense dreams and night visions, also poetry, storytelling, music, and the arts generally, and, naturally, religion itself. All children manifest most of these behaviors to some degree, but we are speaking here of a

very intense level indeed—the examples that follow make this clear—
and, moreover, one which prolongs itself beyond childhood into adult
life.

Some psychic individuals develop into visionary artists (the close
connections between psychic ability and the creative arts have been
touched on many times in previous chapters), and we begin with these,
considering specifically William Blake and W. B. Yeats.

William Blake (1757–1827), the remarkable visionary painter and
poet, was born in the heart of crowded London, near what is today
Liverpool Street Station, the son of lower middle-class parents engaged
in haberdashery. The family was all religiously inclined, but in an altogether normal way. Blake's psychic visions began early.[1] It is said that
he had his first vision of God, peering in at him through the window, at
the age of four, which frightened him badly. Subsequently more detailed
visions were received by him joyfully, though not so by his family. At
the age of "eight or ten," when walking on Peckham Rye, he saw a tree
filled with angels. On another occasion he saw angels walking among
haymakers at work. We note, incidentally, that though born in the heart
of London, Blake was drawn irresistibly as a youngster to the countryside of south London. "Everything that lives is holy," he said often
throughout his life.[2]

Blake's elder brother, James, also had something of William's visionary gifts. "He had his spiritual and visionary side too; he would at times
talk Swedenborg, talking of seeing Abraham and Moses."[3] Again we
see the psychic tendency running in a family. Many regarded William
as mad throughout his life, a slur commonly cast upon psychics and
visionaries. James was also thought to be mad, but quietly mad, whereas
William was described as wild and stormy.

Blake's "premature" talent as an artist emerged in his earliest
years, and at the age of ten he was sent to art school. Poetry came
somewhat later, but he was already producing fine work in early adolescence. Outright paranormal abilities were also apparent. Following
art school, he was to be apprenticed to an engraver and to this end was
taken to be interviewed by the engraver to the King, a Mr. Rylands.

After the interview Blake said that he disliked the man's face and that "it looks as if he will live to be hanged." Rylands was hanged twelve years later for a forgery on the East India Dock Company.[4]

W. B. Yeats (1865–1939), likewise a major visionary poet and painter, was born in Dublin, Ireland. His grandfather had been a clergyman, but his father was a total skeptic. As a youngster, though "brilliant" at school subjects, Yeats was shy and dreamy,[5] "addicted to reverie," and intensely religious, saying his prayers devoutly every evening.[6] Richard Ellman further writes:

> When he was fifteen, the awakening of sex, which came upon him "like the bursting of a shell" made his dreams so attractive that he wanted to be alone with them, and slept in a cave or among the rhododendrons and rocks of Howth Castle. . . . He was fascinated above all by his childish image of the magician, an image which is common enough in boyhood but which took hold of him with peculiar force.[7]

At the age of eighteen "his daydreaming continued unabated" and he remained in fact a lifelong mystic. At one stage he was a member of the Theosophists under Madame Blavatsky, but left to become a member of the rather more infamous Hermetic Students of the Golden Dawn.

> Unlike Madame Blavatsky, who continually warned her followers against the dangers of performing "phenomena," the chiefs of the Golden Dawn encouraged members to demonstrate their powers over the material universe . . . early in his acquaintance with Mathers, the magician put the Tantric symbol of fire against his forehead, and Yeats shortly perceived a huge Titan rising from desert sands. He was greatly excited . . . and he soon found that he could obtain even more remarkable results by trying Mather's methods with others, especially with sensitive women . . . he put a death symbol on the forehead of William Sharp, who without having seen the symbol immediately thought he saw a hearse passing outside.[8]

An example of an outstanding British medium is Ena Twigg. She was born in Gillingham, Kent, in a lower middle-class family that she describes as "typically English." Though not specially religious, all the family were psychic to some degree, although in general the others resisted the impulses, finding them an irritation, even an oppression.

From a very early age Ena found herself surrounded by what she calls "the misty people." The name arises from the fact that the figures in question are transparent. These and other unusual events in Ena's life did not, however, cause her any problems.

> No one at school or at home thought me eccentric or peculiar—and on the surface I was quite a normal little English girl. I never talked about my "misty people" to grown-ups, and so I was left alone to visit and chat and play with them. They were my best friends, and if sometimes my mother or Nanny caught me talking to them—why, many children have imaginary playmates, so they did not take the matter seriously. Of course, the people I played with were not visible to other people, but there was nothing odd about them to me. They didn't seem imaginary—they seemed quite real. There were grown-ups and children as in the real world. . . . I cannot remember a time when I wasn't psychic. I discovered when I was only about two or three that I could fly upstairs and downstairs after my body had been put to bed. It was very amusing. I could see and hear what the grown-ups were doing over their cups of tea . . . as a tiny child all this seemed natural to me, and it was some time before I discovered that there was anything unique or unusual about it.[9]

As a child, then, Ena also had what are usually called "out-of-the-body" experiences. Many psychic adults have them, but it is rare in a very young child. Ena has gone on to realize her gifts in remarkable ways, as we already saw in chapter 9.

Mrs. W. D., to whose story we now come, is almost certainly an example of a repressed psychic, one whose fantasy life as a child was so badly hampered that the faculty "went underground" only to emerge in middle life after a nervous crisis that stopped short only of actual breakdown.

As a child Mrs. D. was intensely attracted to the fairy world in all its respects (as indeed she still is). Far from such interest being tolerated, or even capitalized upon, it was instead crushed under a rigid, conventional religious upbringing. But every moment spent in church was hateful to the child; instead she "talked to the trees" and at night before she slept journeyed on a magic carpet among the blue stars.

Following this unsatisfactory upbringing, her adolescence was normal and rather successful. Mrs. D. trained as an opera singer and was set to take up a professional career, when she married and decided, after a struggle with herself, that she would settle down to married life and help her husband run his guest house. Apart from her operatic gifts, Mrs. D. was also a keen amateur painter, good enough later to have canvases accepted for the Royal Academy Summer Exhibition. Interestingly, Mrs. D. sometimes now paints with her left hand, and also when she has to lift some heavy object one-handed (say, when cooking) she instinctively employs her left rather than her right hand. On this basis alone we can assume that Mrs. D. was a natural left-hander who was forced to use her right hand (like those individuals already encountered in chapter 11)—yet further evidence of the repressive nature of her upbringing. Mrs. D.'s latent left-handedness is confirmed in the "twirling" behavior she indulged in after her breakthrough to her psychic self. She twirled to the left. (She had no idea of the significance of this directional movement until I explained it to her.)

In middle life, her husband died, leaving her in sole charge of the guest house, which she ran throughout the period of her breakthrough and still runs successfully to this day. Following the death of her husband, and also for personal reasons that she does not want publicized, Mrs. D. now drifted into a long period of gradually intensifying clinical depression. (However, although the word "clinical" is used here, Mrs. D. did not in fact seek any form of psychotherapy or psychiatric counseling.) She writes:

My being was somehow removed to a strange land, where (I) with little ego left stood apart, looking at a world of ghosts. I was lost. Then followed a period of great distress and tears that fell, just fell from my eyes in cascades, like the flow from a tap. This condition lasted for weeks. . . .

During this period of intense sorrow I took no food at all for several weeks, only liquid, black coffee and brandy, and sixty or more cigarettes a day. My stomach would not accept food. There was no hunger, I had no hunger.

I continued nevertheless to run my guest house, and paradoxically had plenty of energy despite little or no sleep, and of course no food. Then the intensity of the sorrow diminished somewhat, and there came a period of simply "not being," of not having an ego. There was still a deep despair, but it had no anchor, it was just a thing in space. The next stage was a still more complete non-being. For example, there was no saliva to swallow, because there was no throat to swallow it with. At this time I recall leaning over the back of a settee and "vanishing." Subsequently I looked in the mirror, and *there was no image,* just a blank mirror. This was good, I thought, I must be dead, or nearly so.

The incident just described was the crisis or turning point of Mrs. D's breakthrough. She had at that moment *become* the mirror image. She had become her alternative, denied unconscious self.[10] The word "breakdown" is totally inappropriate, for as we see in a moment, the outcome of the experience is wholly and dramatically additive, and in no way at all subtractive or diminishing.

I sat down in a big armchair, lay back and relaxed. Suddenly I was enveloped in a bright, bright and intensely white light. I seemed suddenly to have been lifted into another world. The tears began to pour in cascades down my face, neck and chest: but I made no sound of crying or sobbing. I suddenly realized that I had *no problems, no problems, no problems.* This was an amazing thought to have after all the shattering sorrow I had experienced, along with every form of negative feeling towards others—bitterness, jealousy, hatred, rage—and of course the feeling of nonexistence. In an instant this vast army of negative feelings and experiences vanished. They seemed to have been swept away by my tears, never to return again. In their place suddenly appeared the bliss of "no problem" and a sudden surge of love of all and everything, all people, all life.

From this point Mrs. D.'s life and being took on the positive (and magical) qualities that have not so much marked as illumined her life since. One more technical detail should be mentioned: Following the long spell of starvation Mrs. D. went to see her doctor. He advised her that her physical condition was extremely precarious and that without a proper intake of food she would die. Overriding her vegetarian objections, he insisted that for the time being she must eat meat and fish. This she did, despite her inner loathing, and as she admits, it did the trick. Her metabolism returned rapidly to normal.

Mrs. D's subsequent experiences recall vividly those of Blake, and as with Blake her visions were followed by the reemergence of painting and, for the first time, poetry. Moving out into the world again, Mrs. D. writes:

I saw rainbow colours everywhere, the trees studded with bright jewels, golden light surrounding objects, with my eyes wide open. These experiences brought also a sense of great joy, a feeling of warmth, love of all and everything, a one-ness with objects animate and inanimate, the love of a stone, a speck of dust on a sunbeam, a twig, the stars, moon and sun. With eyes closed there would be fantastic colours, always brighter, clearer colours, many, many archways, so beautiful golden archways studded with precious stones of many hues. The light was very bright, of an intensity that one could read by, as it were, and sometimes this light would also fill a dark room where I sat. I did not realize then that the light was within me, not in the room. What a superb experience it was. It lasted for many weeks. I thought I was in fairyland, and no one knew about it, it was my very own magic land.

Now she walked on air. All her senses were alive as never before—especially the sense of smell. (Sometimes, as she admits, her senses fooled her. One day she rejoiced that she could already smell the scent of roses on a bush she saw in the distance. But this turned out to be some other shrub with pink flowers that had no scent at all. Clearly, like Ruth, Mrs. D. could now create her own reality.) She painted rapidly and furiously, almost continuously, "vast quantities of technically bad pictures, but they expressed the inner state." When she was not painting, she wrote quantities of poetry and poetic prose. There was much laughter in this period, and a sense of happiness that brought tears of joy to her eyes. Securing the doors from sudden invasion by her clients, she would dance and twirl through her apartment in her newfound delight. She felt herself to be almost magical. When she needed to check something in a book, for example, she would grab the book and fling it open—and find it to be open at the page she needed.

After this heady time, she began to read widely and to look for answers to what had happened to her. She began studying both esoteric religions and disciplines and equally scientific works of psychology and physiology. Nowhere, however, could she find any adequate answer. She was and is absolutely convinced that the explanation of her experience has nothing to do with religion (though many people, of course, would have felt they had had a religious revelation), but is physiological–psychological. Fringe religions at least agree that the phenomena exist, even though their explanations fail to satisfy the deeply questioning individual. Psychology does not even acknowledge the phenomena except as the incoherent by-product of mental illness. But the experiences of Mrs. D. and others are not incoherent.

In fact Mrs. D. exhibited many of the major features of schizophrenia, without actually having the illness. She was too old for schizophrenia for one thing (see chapter 15), but more importantly, she never lost touch with reality. She continued to run a busy guest house without any break—and what is still more, no one noted any oddness in her day-to-day behavior. It would be quite impossible for a real schizophrenic to go undetected in these circumstances. The question for academic psychology, then, is how is it possible to have schizophrenia without having it? Mediums and other psychics also hear disembodied voices and see visions: they, too, are not mentally ill.

Another important question arises at this point: where does the intelligent psychic individual in crisis go for help and understanding? Religion is of no use, nor is psychiatry, as will become clear in a moment.

The most startling feature of Mrs. D.'s experiences over the past ten years, however, has still not been mentioned. In her search for information she joined a number of fringe organizations and took part in their activities. One of these was an "absent healing" group. In such groups those present concentrate their thoughts on some selected person who is ill, in an effort to aid that person's recovery. On the first occasion in which Mrs. D. participated, she was abruptly seized by a sudden "force." She slid to the ground, moaning and gasping, and describing, in the first person, the symptoms of the woman the group was trying to heal (but of which she had no conscious knowledge—she knew only the woman's name). She said: "I cannot breathe, I am choking, my side will not move," and so on. The woman in question had had a stroke, was paralyzed, and had great difficulty in breathing and speaking. In addition to experiencing the physical symptoms, Mrs. D. also mentally saw herself in some kind of college with a group of students. The woman had in fact been warden of a college and had suffered a stroke following problems with one of the male students. After recovering from this experience, Mrs. D., though reluctant, was persuaded on two subsequent occasions to take part in this group's activities. On both occasions the same phenomenon occurred. She found herself suffering the physical symptoms of the sick person, at the same time seeing a vision of the sick person with significant detail. After these experiences, however, Mrs. D. was only revived with difficulty. They were clearly dangerous for her. She then refused to undergo any further experimentation and has attempted nothing of this kind since.

So, to repeat the question: to whom does a person like Mrs. D. turn for help and understanding? From scientists she will receive only indulgent contempt. Psychiatrists will tell her only that she is mentally disturbed. Priests and clergymen will trot out their tired, unhelpful formulas.

The problem involved is underlined by another striking case, that of Mrs. E. C., who contacted me recently. She is a graduate in mathematics and a teacher, married, and with a family. She had a strict Catholic upbringing, and from this developed an almost crippling sense of guilt, regarding herself as a sinner. If she stole a cake, for example, as children will, she would be tormented with guilt, would say penitential prayers for months on end, and be unable to sleep. She soon formed the idea that she must belong to the devil. Instead of growing out of such childish fears and imaginings, she found them reinforced by what began happening to her as a young adult, and there has been no change with increasing age. She began to become aware which people around her would die, and when, and in what manner.

This perhaps sounds altogether ridiculous, until one begins to hear her evidence. For example, a neighbor's mother died, on a Sunday. The man was very upset. Mrs. C. found herself thinking, "Won't it be sad for him when his wife dies next Sunday—oh, no—that would be too soon, that would be awful—no, she'll die a year from now, on a Sunday." Sure enough, the wife did die a year later and indeed on a Sunday. Another neighbor was in the habit of scolding her son excessively. Mrs. C. thought, "She doesn't deserve to have such a good son, it would serve her right if he was killed on his bike." A couple of months later the boy was killed on his bicycle by a car.

Mrs. C. was visiting her psychiatrist, to whom she had turned for help with her problem. He, as usual, was urging her to "face the devil" or "test the devil." He was in the habit of proposing that she experimentally choose someone for death, in the clear belief that the test would fail, and that Mrs. C.'s "fantasy" would be undermined. (However, Mrs. C. cannot control the thoughts that come into her head. At this point she became aware of a passenger airliner flying past overhead. "Oh dear," she thought. "I do hope that plane isn't going to fly into a line and crash." A few days later she read in her newspaper that an airliner in India had hit a telegraph line and crashed. A few days after that she was driving her car behind a travel coach of Court Line. The phrase "Court Line" reminded her of "caught in a line." "Oh," she thought. "I hope that doesn't mean another plane is going to crash." Next day her newspaper headline read "Court Line Crashes." The travel firm had gone bankrupt.

This last example is impressive because it clearly displays the punning or associative thinking that is so typical of the unconscious mind. Psychoanalysis in particular uses free verbal association to track down the source of patients' problems. (For further discussion of these matters see earlier books.[11])

It is the *mass* of examples that Mrs. C. produces that helps convince one that she is speaking the truth, plus the fact that she is close to tears when telling of these incidents. She has been having psychoanalysis for *seventeen years* in an attempt to halt her strange and unwanted thoughts, but with no success.

One of the reasons—perhaps the basic reason—for the nonsuccess of Mrs. C.'s therapy is that the psychiatrist does not believe her, i.e., he does not believe it is possible to have real premonitions. All the individual pursued by psychic events needs to be told by some such clown (I cannot bring myself to use a milder word)—a hard-line psychiatrist, a hard-line physicist, or whatever—is that it is not happening. That is enough to drive the person into complete desperation (as happened with Carlotta Moran). An acceptance of the phenomena as genuine would be the first step to persuading Mrs. C. to understand that she does not *cause* the deaths, which is what she in fact believes. The paranormal universe is non-causal, or rather, a-causal.[12]

Seeing a future event does not cause it to happen. (Science, of course, has no intention of agreeing to the existence of any alternative *a-causal* framework of meaningful events.)

In conclusion here are some of my own experiences of the inner alternative world of the mind.

Some people reach this inner world by holding themselves just on the edge of sleep after going to bed at night. Others, myself included (and, for example, Swedenborg), reach it by remaining on the threshold of waking in the morning.

A typical entry into the inner world for me might be as follows. I become aware that I am almost awake and mentally decline to wake further. Suddenly I begin to feel myself move. The movement appears wholly real and literal. I may dive backwards, head first, through the pillow and down through the floor and soon am in rapid free fall. Often a strong roaring, rushing noise accompanies this descent. It may last for minutes. Sometimes it ends in falling asleep (the pun here is intentional: why in fact do we use the phrase "falling asleep"?). But if I am lucky the fall through empty, semi-black space is now streaked with brilliant colors, or sometimes with spinning, glowing points of light of all possible hues. Then I may land, with a little bump. I may land on a concrete surface against a wall with a door in it, or on the floor of a cellar with a passageway leading off. When I get up and go through the door, or the passage, I am in the magic world. Or sometimes I simply snap into the magical universe in mid-fall without further ado. Or again, sometimes I can just be there, suddenly without falling at all.

The inner universe of which I now partake, with, what is more, the full consciousness of being myself, and of being *there*, takes myriad forms. I might be running through a beautiful countryside, delighting in the air, the sunshine, and the sights and sounds of nature. Then perhaps I come to, or start off in, a town. Here the architecture is of an amazing beauty and variety. Yet there is prosaic life too. There will be streets of shops and cafés, with many people in them. It is all full of interest, all totally new and unexpected. It is as if I were really in a modern, Western equivalent of the Arabian nights. Yet the best part of all is the triumphant feeling of being there, of having escaped from all the cares and limitations of the daily human grind, of being in my own personal wonderland where all is possible, and where the imagination can never be exhausted. I talk to the people. I may meet a girl, and with luck, go to bed with her. The sex is not just as good as, but better than that obtainable in the real world, because one's own personal archetypal wishes and fantasies may be, and often are, lived out.

The phrase "may be" is important, however. For the people of this inner world are by no means just one's puppets (any more than Ruth's hallucinations were in chapter 10). One has to relate to them, like any real people. Nevertheless, one's position is privileged. I know that the others are my own creation, in some sense, even though they are of the unconscious, not the conscious, mind.

On other occasions the inner universe is not at all like any normal world. Sometimes one hangs in space, as it were, and an endless series of paintings, drawings, or tableaux is presented to me, or sometimes an orchestra will play. The beauty and creative stature of these various art forms is absolutely breathtaking and genuine. One's mind reels before the achievements one is shown—oh, if only one could bring them back into the everyday world. Creative artists do, of course, bring back a tiny part of this inexhaustible hoard for us to enjoy in our daylight hours. This, at least, is no fairy gold. It is real and genuine.

Sometimes again, printed matter will float before my eyes—a newspaper, with every word, headline and column sharply in focus, or a book, perhaps full of exquisite illustrations, or poetry. I am always eager to read this material, but one has to be careful not to get too interested or excited, because one can suddenly find oneself awake. (Coleridge, we remember, woke up before he could finish *Kubla Khan*.) On closer examination the material might be made up of nonsense syllables—ug noo tomera pin nosa'—page after page of it, all neatly and beautifully printed. What compositor is setting up these blocks of print? At other times the script may be Arabic or Chinese. I have no idea if this is genuine—it looks genuine. On other occasions I will be reading a novel—not any novel consciously known to me—but as yet I have never managed to read one of these beyond a few pages. Is one here raiding the storehouse that is drawn upon in automatic writing—already set up and awaiting publication?

(What is the point in evolutionary terms of this inexhaustible treasure house that all possess but most never visit? Perhaps its purpose is ultimately to turn mankind from an imprisoning, because purely material, future. Christ, after all, said the kingdom of heaven is within us.)

Then there are the dreams that are closer to what most people understand by dreaming. When I was younger these took the form of long adventures or mystery stories—of a life before the mast, the career of a spy, and whatever. These stories lasted most of the night (as do their present counterparts). I can be aware of having ceased to dream in the normal nightly cycle of the brain's rhythms, and then resume, and even wake fully, then sleep again, whereupon the story picks up smoothly and effortlessly once more, rather like a film that has been stopped for an interval. These stories or films in which one played the leading part were every whit as good as any first-class media product, for which in the waking state one willingly pays hard-earned money. No, far better, because I was playing the lead myself.

Now that I am not so young, the character of these dreams has deepened remarkably. As before, they can last an entire night, and continue through one or more waking periods. But now I will live, say, the apparently true life-cycle of a child in a northern mill town of the last century, or the childhood of an individual who is to become a great composer.

These lives, far more real than any memory, are lived firsthand and with total immediacy. Yet somehow my own nondreaming mind is also present, watching. So I not only live the child's (or it can be an adult's) life with full immediacy, but can see the beauty amidst the ugliness, the poetry amidst the despair, and the otherwise pathetic or tragic. If I am, say, a to-be composer, or writer, or whatever, I grasp how this childhood kiss, or this run of horses, will one day be transmuted into music or poetry.

There is no call to take my word alone on the sheer mechanics of the artistic, transmuting process just described. This same transformation can be observed in the work of every artist, poet, composer. Among poets, perhaps Dylan Thomas has shown it at its clearest; but all show it, and some have talked of it. The novelist Margaret Kennedy writes in her book *The Constant Nymph* as follows.[13] (Lewis is a composer.)

"When I was a boy," said Lewis abruptly, "I used to sleep out on some cliffs in Cornwall. And there were some birds, whole flocks of them, I d-don't know what they were, used to fly out to sea just before it got light. I remember I woke up once, when the moon had set and it was quite d-dark, and all the air was full of them. I couldn't see them. I heard wings. . . ."

Tessa, on the grass at his side, stirred a little in response to the excitement behind his hesitating, drowsy voice. She knew that some impulse had prompted him to tell them of a supreme moment, one of those instants, rare and indescribable, when the quickened imagination stores up an impression which may become a secret key to beauty, the inspiration of a lifetime. Her mind swung back to meet the mind of that lost boy who had lain awake upon a high mysterious cliff, beside a whispering sea. She, too, heard wings.

All creative individuals have some access to the process just described, which my own dreams and those of others like me suggest to be a constant, miraculous process taking place continuously within the unconscious minds of all of us, breaking through to consciousness only sporadically in the human beings we call artists. Current academic psychology has, of course, no explanation whatsoever to offer of the creative process or of art itself.

On my early mornings I awake awestruck, dazed, and transformed by the events through which I have lived that night. It is not simply a matter of mere events, arresting though they can be. It is the sense of affect (emotion), the insight into the working of a mind, of "someone else's" mind, as well as my own.

For an hour or more, on waking, I wander back through the new life I have just lived. And it will stay with me through the day, another chapter from an inexhaustible dream volume. So many, many personalities contained within each human being, like the millions of eggs in a single fish. And most of us only realize and live just one of them. Yet each of us, I believe, can potentially reach and actualize that inner store. (Some practical suggestions as to precisely how have been given in my earlier books.[14])

The foregoing material, and indeed the whole of this book, exposes as complete nonsense the standard scientific view of dreams as some kind of poisonous or incoherent by-product of normal consciousness. The typical views of Francis Crick, an establishment scientist and Nobel Prize winner, are especially pathetic.[15] He considers dreams to be a process whereby useless mental material picked up during the day is disposed of by the brain. He writes in conclusion: "the practice of remembering dreams should be discouraged." How well this statement reveals the desperate, frozen paranoia of the Western scientist toward dreams and the unconscious generally. In this area modern science can justifiably be said to be both repressive and fascist—that is, psychologically disturbed and politically despicable.[16] It was, essentially, this same attitude that led to the burning and torturing of so many unfortunate wretches who dared in former times to proclaim the validity of our human "secret life."

It seems clear, at any rate, that all stories and legends like those of Aladdin's cave, of fairyland, of enchantment and bewitchment, are really in origin descriptions of trips to the inner universe—which those who experienced them believed to be objectively real. Swedenborg, the outstanding mystic and psychic, believed that he literally traveled to the scene of the afterlife that awaits us beyond death, and wrote of it in detail in his book *Heaven and Hell*. Swedenborg, incidentally, had earlier published a collection of his dreams, some of which were of a grossly sexual nature.

Artists and psychics alike share a ready access to the unconscious mind. They will almost certainly as children have given indications of their gift—perhaps by seeing visions, or perhaps by a more than usually intense interest in nature, or in stories of the imagination, which goes well beyond the normal. I myself, though I saw no visions, was, like William Blake and Martyn Pryer, in love with nature, and, like Mrs. D., totally fascinated by every form of magical story and legend. When adolescence came I had to hide these latter "childish" interests from my school friends, but at the age of fourteen I was still methodically searching junk shops, looking for a real magic carpet or a wishing ring. The song "Somewhere Over the Rainbow" made me weep for the magical world that I was sure existed, but from which I was shut out. Yet, in the end, I found it.

In a sane and properly balanced society, youngsters such as those we have described would be trained to develop and apply their magical gifts and to teach others less gifted how they might also achieve them. That day may perhaps come.

17

BUT WHERE
IN THE BRAIN IS THE
UNC⊕NSCI⊕US?

We should probably never finally close the door on the possibility of discarnate or spirit beings existing independently of ourselves. To do so would be arrogant.

However, with that cautionary note and despite the dramatic evidence of apparently discarnate entities or forces noisily breaking up rooms, starting fires, attacking and severely bruising human beings, and causing some of them to burst into flames, we have, nevertheless, throughout this book seen persuasive evidence that these entities or forces are directly associated with, and indeed are directly *produced* by, certain individuals. We have considered an unbroken chain of evidence leading from the minor neurotic behaviors of everyday life (which in themselves are, of course, already clear evidence of an activity of mind at least partly independent of normal consciousness) to the ultimate and sometimes terrifying experience of the incubus and the poltergeist, the raging play of temporarily uncontrollable forces. In short, these macabre events appear to be the result of some kind of externalization of energies latent within the human personality, currently not understood.

The self-governing part of the human mind that can function independently of normal consciousness (more so or less so, depending on the precise circumstances) is usually referred to as "the unconscious." This term has been kept in the present book. It is nevertheless an unfortunate one—for the unconscious mind is not necessarily unconscious *of itself*, it is only (as a rule) unconscious to normal waking consciousness. A better name for the unconscious would be "alternative consciousness," a name that rightly suggests the separate identity, autonomy, and "own logic" activity of this biological and psychological phenomenon.

Theoretically, it is possible to consider that the "unconscious" mind is not located, or at any rate not wholly located, in the physical brain. Some outstanding modern psychologists (such as Sir John Eccles) do not consider that even the conscious mind can be wholly reduced to a supporting physiological structure. Nevertheless, the extreme view that the unconscious mind has no location of any kind in the physical brain would be a giant philosophical assumption, one that, following Occam's principle of economy, we ought to avoid until and unless we are forced to accept it. Even the more modest assumption that the unconscious mind may not be entirely linked to a physiological underpinning is not the one we should start with. We must begin with the assumption that the unconscious mind does have an identifiable physical seat somewhere in the nervous system.

It is a remarkable circumstance that neither Freud nor Jung, nor any subsequent psychoanalyst or psychiatrist, ever made a concerted attempt to identify the physical basis of the unconscious mind—which, as a concept and a reality, they were nevertheless totally prepared to defend with their professional lives. Why did, and do, psychoanalysts and psychiatrists duck the issue of the physical basis of the unconscious?

Their reason is both a strength and a weakness. First, psychological events, of which unconscious contents are one form, exist in their own right. They *exist,* quite independently of whether or not a physiological basis can be found for them. Even if such a basis is found, the psychological events concerned cannot be *reduced* to the physical events. Psychological events are an independent and higher order phenomenon. They exist in their own right.

From one point of view, then, psychoanalysts are perfectly justified in refusing to fight on a physiological battleground. But to refuse to be *forced* to fight on a physiological battleground is one thing. To refuse to enter that battleground voluntarily and "without prejudice" (as the legal phrase has it) is another. The failure of psychoanalysts to enter the lists on this voluntary basis is not a strength, but a weakness, and a very damaging one to their credibility.

By contrast, the general physical location of the *conscious* mind is rather well established. We know that the cerebral cortex (the outer layers) of the two hemispheres of the cerebrum is heavily involved. Voluntary motor movements are directed by the cerebral cortex, for example, and fairly precise areas have been mapped that, in the normal intact brain, deal specifically with finger movement, eye movement, operations of the mouth and throat in speaking, and so on. We also know what areas of the normal intact cerebral cortex are principally concerned in producing language, in working out mathematical problems, in analyzing visual stimuli, and so on. Despite a marked tendency (in the opinion of some of us) for academic psychologists to oversimplify the problems involved, there is no doubt that in broad general terms the cerebral cortex is, in some sense, the home of much of the activity we call waking consciousness.

The purpose of this chapter is to show that the unconscious mind, too, does have an identifiable physiological basis. Where, then, is it?

There are really only three possibilities. The first is that the unconscious mind is somehow interwoven with, or adjacent to, the conscious mind in the cerebral cortex. Here the front-running theory of recent times is that the so-called minor of the two cerebral hemispheres (the right one) is the seat of the unconscious. A second possibility is that the unconscious mind is housed in the less evolved or "primitive" centers of the lower brain—the thalamus, the hypothalamus, the reticular system, the limbic system, and so on. A third possibility is that the unconscious mind is located in the cerebellum.

THE RIGHT (MINOR) CEREBRAL HEMISPHERE AS THE HOME OF THE UNCONSCIOUS

Psychologists had long suspected that the two cerebral hemispheres of the human brain monitored different cognitive functions. The dramatic final proof that this was indeed so came in the early 1960s with the development of a brain operation designed to treat chronic, progressive epilepsy. In this operation the corpus callosum, a body of complex fibers joining the two halves of the cerebrum, is cut completely through. The two cerebral hemispheres are then internally isolated one from another.

The study of patients who had had this operation confirmed that the left (major) cerebral hemisphere (governing the right side of the body) dealt with language functions, writing, arithmetical calculation, and so on, in about 90 percent of people. In most people the right (minor) hemisphere is concerned with spatial relationships and drawing.

There is no doubt that in the intact brain of the normal adult each of the two hemispheres specializes in certain functions—nor can it be disputed that following the corpus callosum operation the individuals concerned exhibit various mental lacks and confusions. If a picture of an everyday object is flashed to the right hemisphere, the person cannot name it, whereas if it is flashed to the left hemisphere, he can. A male patient reported, following the operation, that he would find himself pulling up his trousers with one hand, while pulling them down with the other. A female patient reported that she would decide on a green dress to wear, but find herself putting on a red one, or discover that she was wearing several pairs of panties.

A number of writers (mainly "fringe" writers but including the psychologist Robert Ornstein[1]) began claiming that the right (minor) hemisphere was the unconscious mind. They cited experiments in which pictures of nudes were shown to the patients' right hemisphere, whereupon the subjects would grin or blush, but be unable to say why. However, the claimants overlooked the fact that the patients *also* equally smiled or blushed when the pictures were shown to the left hemisphere—though this time the patients were able to say why.

The argument that the right hemisphere represents the unconscious mind falls down on three major counts. The first is that in the normal brain, where the corpus callosum is intact, the two sides of the cerebrum have no secrets from each other. Any information processed or stored in one hemisphere is instantly available to the other. Something like 15,000 messages a second flash across the connecting corpus callosum.[2] The position is really rather like a company with two offices, in the same block on the same floor, where in each, for convenience, two types of activity are segregated. But any information known in one office is instantly available to the other, simply by touching an intercom.

More telling still are the results obtained from a different surgical operation: one complete hemisphere (either the minor or the major) is totally removed, to combat cancer or some other malignant tumor. Many dozens of operations for complete removal of the major left hemisphere have been performed on right-handed children. All such children soon begin to develop in the remaining minor right hemisphere all the functions alleged to be the exclusive property of the other—speech, arithmetical ability, and so on.[3] The youngest person ever to have this operation was a three-week-old baby—so there was no question of the minor hemisphere merely mimicking functions already developed by the major hemisphere. In this case the minor hemisphere had to undertake all functions from scratch. As an adult of twenty-one years the person concerned showed no psychological or motor defects at all.[4]

In those who undergo complete removal of one or other hemisphere as adults recovery is slower, and some deficit remains, due to the general loss of plasticity of older organisms. But none of the adults whose major hemisphere was removed became the speechless vegetable that the surgeons initially feared.[5] Speech and arithmetical functions began to develop as soon as the post-operative shock was over. Perhaps even more striking is the fact that no child or adult who has undergone complete removal of either hemisphere has ever shown any physical paralysis or impairment of motor function on the "missing" side of the body.[6]

Some individuals with a genetic defect are born without any corpus callosum at all. As adults these individuals show almost none of the performance deficits and confusions of adults whose corpus callosum has been cut. It is again clear that, when the corpus callosum is absent from birth, both sides of the brain develop *all* functions independently.

Mainstream psychologists now agree that the minor hemisphere of the patient who has undergone corpus callosum surgery is not unconscious at all. It is conscious, but it is not verbal; it simply cannot express itself in words. In the normal person with corpus callosum intact, however, there is not the slightest question of the minor hemisphere being unconscious. The two hemispheres, working together, make up and *are* the conscious, cognitive mind.

The third type of evidence is equally conclusive. If the minor hemisphere in the intact person were indeed the unconscious mind, or even had a special relationship with the unconscious, there are several consequences that must follow and that are readily testable. One is that the electrical activity of the brain associated with dreaming ought to show up exclusively in the minor hemisphere, or at least be more marked in the minor hemisphere. This is not the case. Both hemispheres show the same activity, and equally intense activity. Further, the biologist and physicist C. Maxwell Cade has developed an instrument he calls the Mind Mirror, which monitors and displays activity in the cerebral brain when meditation is taking place. Once again, meditation should favor the minor hemisphere, if this were indeed in any sense the location of the unconscious mind. But again both hemispheres show the same activity, and equal amounts of the same activity.

There are two types of conditioned response that the human nervous system acquires. One is Pavlovian conditioning, and the other is Skinnerian conditioning. The Pavlovian variety has to do with states of emotion, involuntary movements, and the autonomic system generally; the Skinnerian with cognitive activity, voluntary movements, and the central nervous system generally. The two kinds of conditioning are absolutely distinct—and indeed their very existence is a powerful argument for the basic duality of the human mind and personality.

Now, if the minor cerebral hemisphere had any kind of link with the "emotional" and unconscious mind, or the autonomic system, which we know to be very closely associated with the unconscious mind, then it would be possible to induce Pavlovian conditioning by electrical stimulation of the minor hemisphere. No such conditioning can be induced by stimulating any part of the minor hemisphere, nor by stimulating any part of the cerebrum whatsoever; nor, further, can any autonomic response as such be reflexively induced in the body by stimulating either hemisphere of the cerebrum. Pavlovian conditioning, however, *can* be achieved by electrical stimulation of the cerebellum, as can the reflex triggering of autonomic functions—two striking pieces of evidence in favor of the close connection of the cerebellum with the unconscious.

In short, then, the proposal that the minor cerebral hemisphere is the seat of the unconscious mind fails and has failed to stand up to experimental investigation. Mainstream psychology no longer argues this position, if indeed it ever did. It is only popular writers on the fringe of professional psychology who are still, unfortunately, attempting to maintain this particular fiction.

THE LOWER BRAIN AS THE UNCONSCIOUS

The idea that the many mid- and lower-brain centers taken together might constitute the seat of the unconscious mind falls on one crucial consideration. Complex and highly evolved though some of these lower centers are, they are nevertheless insufficiently evolved and insufficiently complex to produce (for example) the rounded and articulate personalities we find speaking through the entranced medium (see chapter 9), the creative and complex content of automatic writing and painting (chapter 5), and of hypnotic regression (chapter 7), or the visual miracles of the "alternative universe" (chapter 16). For the production, sustaining and elaboration of such material we require an extremely large and *massively* complex organ, such as the cerebrum and its cerebral cortex.

The lower centers of the brain function principally as way stations, examining, refining, distributing, and amplifying the mass of basic sensory information not only continuously pouring in from the outside world, but also arising within the body itself, before passing the information on to still higher centers.

This information passes ultimately to the cerebral cortex (as well as independently to the cerebellum) and until it arrives there does not become conscious. The experimental blocking (by electrical impulses) of signals at any of the lower levels, right up to the level of the cortex, prevents the signal from proceeding farther and thus from becoming conscious.

One of the effects of LSD and other such drugs (as we saw in chapter 7) is effectively to generate false information in lower centers (such as the pineal gland), which is then passed on as if it had been received as genuine sensory information.

What can be conceded without argument, however, is that much of the energy of the unconscious (and, for that matter, of the conscious mind also) is derived from the lower centers. Striking evidence of this claim is provided by kundalini meditation[7] in which the adept subjectively experiences a rush of energy passing up the spinal cord and bursting into the conscious brain as a dazzling white light. This subjective experience of energy has, however, a very real objective correlate—for sometimes nerves and nerve centers are damaged by its passing.[8] Or again, the reticular activating system, an organization of the lower brain centers, is responsible for flooding the body and the higher brain with energy, arousing the cerebral cortex to maximum alertness whenever danger threatens.

Probably, too, though this is speculation rather than experimentally demonstrated fact, the unstructured nightmare that swamps us in some nameless and inchoate terror or loathing derives its impulse and energy from the lower centers. Such a nightmare is simply the welling up of primitive fear from some of the oldest levels of our being—from what has been correctly described as our reptilian brain (the brain our distant ancestors evolved long ago, in the Jurassic age and earlier).

The incubus attack or ghoulish seizure, however, as we have seen, shows the wealth of elaboration, precise detail, and continuity that only the highest evolved levels of the nervous system are capable of supporting. Energy is one thing: elaboration is quite another.

THE CEREBELLUM AS THE UNCONSCIOUS

The cerebellum, an apparently much smaller object than the cerebrum (the organ that we usually and chauvinistically refer to as "the brain"), lies at the back and base of the skull, behind the spinal cord, squeezed down into a forgotten corner, by reason mainly of the dramatic growth in recent evolutionary time of the apparently much larger cerebrum.

Yet the appearances here are wholly deceptive. The cerebellum (which, very like the cerebrum, has two hemispheres and a cortex) possesses by reason of its deep, walnut-like fissures a surface area *three-quarters as great as that of the cerebrum.* "Surface area" equals cortex. The cerebellum, then, possesses three quarters as much cortex as the cerebrum.[9]

By reason of its position and apparent smallness, the cerebellum is easily overlooked, and it is, indeed, totally overlooked by modern psychology. "Totally overlooked" is a very strong statement, but justification of it is only too easy to come by, and we make a brief detour for that purpose.

At the time of writing (which happened to be the start of the university academic year) the textbooks on offer to students at the London University Bookshop were examined. One or more of these texts (depending on the precise recommendations of course tutors) becomes the student's bible for the three years of his undergraduate course. These books, it must be emphasized, are written by pillars of the psychological establishment: to be commissioned to write such a standard text, with its financial and other rewards, is one of the perks earned by a lifetime's outstanding contribution to the field. The purpose of examining these texts was to establish the number of pages in each devoted to the cerebellum.

Lindzey, Hall, and Thompson's *Psychology* has 2 pages on the cerebellum out of a total of 762 pages. Smith and Sarason's *Psychology: The Frontiers of Behaviour* has 2 out of 658 pages. Hilgard and Atkinson's *Introduction to Psychology* has 2 out of 587. McConnell's *Understanding Human Behaviour* has 1 out of 780. These four books are typical. Yet perhaps what we are looking for is in the specialist textbooks of physiological psychology? Carlson's *The Physiology of Behaviour* has 4 pages on the cerebellum out of a total of 690. Thompson's *Foundations of Physiological Psychology* has 7 out of 625. Grossman's *Textbook of Physiological Psychology* has 15 out of 890. Clearly the phrase "totally overlooked" is hardly an exaggeration.

A few dedicated psychologists and neuropsychologists are, nevertheless, working full time on the study of the cerebellum and its role in behavior and personality. It is from them, and from occasional asides in medical and other research papers or books essentially concerned with something else, that we learn something of the astonishing truth about this organ. In considering the known facts about the cerebellum we are forced to conclude that its neglect by modern psychology has been no oversight—and can only be the result of a deep-seated fear of the cerebellum, this major organ that proves in the event to be both Aladdin's lamp and Pandora's box.

For brevity, the attributes of the cerebellum are listed in summary.

1. As already emphasized, though it cannot be overemphasized, the surface area of the cerebellum is actually three quarters that of the cerebrum.

2. Parts of the cerebellum are very new. In the same period of evolutionary time during which the cerebrum and its cortex came to such prominence (the last sixty million years), the cerebellum has also developed the two cerebellar hemispheres it now possesses. The development of these hemispheres has more than doubled the size of the cerebellum.

3. This organ is, therefore, very much an on-going phenomenon, not some evolutionary relic. Parts of it, nevertheless, are very old.

It looks very much in fact as if nature originally intended to make the cerebellum the headquarters of the total nervous system, but then changed its mind and developed the cerebrum instead.[10] The cerebellum, however, was in business on its own account before the cerebrum ever appeared.

4. Nowadays the cerebellum (as all agree) is the headquarters of the autonomic nervous system while the cerebrum is the headquarters of the central nervous system. Thus electrical stimulation of the cerebellum produces a wide range of autonomic responses—decrease in tension in the walls of blood vessels, contraction of the pupil of the eye, and so on. This paramount role of the cerebellum in relation to the autonomic nervous system is of the greatest interest, given the close association of the autonomic system with all the phenomena considered throughout this book. Most importantly, stimulation of the cerebellum also produces the twitches of the mouth, face, and limbs observed in dreaming, and the powerful kicks and other movements we sometimes also make when asleep. Here, then, is strong evidence that the cerebellum is directly involved in the production of the dream itself and perhaps of the dream consciousness.

While modern psychology acknowledges the leadership of the cerebellum in respect of the autonomic system, it at no point considers the cerebellum might possess any form of consciousness, not even of dream consciousness.

5. The cerebellar cortex has, nevertheless, extensive sensory projection areas. That is to say, stimulation of sensory receptors produces an *organized* pattern of projections in the cerebellum, just as it does in the cerebrum. Such sensory projection areas—where informational pathways from the lower centers arrive and simply stop—are believed, in the cerebrum, to be associated with the production of consciousness.[11] Why should they not be associated with the production of consciousness in the cerebellum?

6. One of the most important single facts concerning the cerebellum is that in mammals this organ develops its own separate sen-

sory information pathways, quite distinct from those ascending to the cerebrum. In more primitive animals (reptiles and below) cerebellum and cerebrum share the same pathways. "Coincidentally" with the development of separate pathways, dreaming begins with mammals: reptiles and other lower organisms do not dream. It is very hard indeed to avoid the conclusion that it is the new independence of the cerebellum that has produced the capacity to dream.

Whether or not this is the case, the independence of the cerebellum means that no action of the cerebrum or of waking consciousness can deprive the cerebellum of its sensory information, or otherwise radically interfere with its autonomy.

7. Women have larger cerebella than men. "Coincidentally," women are more involved than men in all the phenomena of this book. Prior to 1983 or so, the claim that women had larger cerebella than men rested on the unreliable dissection of cadavers. Now James Prescott has confirmed this formerly tentative finding using the modern brain scanner.[12]

8. Asiatics have much larger cerebella than Europeans "very incompletely covered by the cerebrum."[13] "Coincidentally," again, we in Europe refer to Asia as "the mystic East."

9. There is twice the incidence of left-handedness among Chinese[14] (figures are lacking for other Asiatic groups) than among Europeans—18 percent as opposed to 9 percent. Is the larger cerebellum responsible for the greater incidence of left-handedness? (In this line of reasoning the problem remains of there being rather fewer left-handed women than men, both in Europe and among Chinese. There ought to be more left-handedness among women and not less, given their larger cerebellum. See chapter 11 for discussion.)

10. The cerebellum itself is left-handed, certainly as regards the cerebrum and waking consciousness.[15] In human beings the two sides of the body are governed by the opposite *cerebral* hemisphere. But in the case of the *cerebellar* hemispheres, the left

hemisphere governs the left side of the body, and the right hemisphere the right side. When cerebrum and cerebellum interact, as they habitually do, nerve impulses between them must cross over in transit.

11. Until recently there was no suggestion in academic psychology that the cerebellum was in any way involved in personality. In 1982, however, the neuropsychologist R. Llinas announced his view that the cerebellum is responsible for the character of our individual handwriting. In demonstrating this proposal on television he programmed a computer with the kinds of neural connections available in the cerebellum. The computer was then able to produce something very much like human handwriting, the first time this effect had been achieved.[16]

    Here then we have a direct link with personality—since graphologists use handwriting to deduce aspects of an individual's personality and emotional character. Not only this, but we here have also at least a tentative link between the cerebellum and automatic writing (see chapter 5).

12. The last statement is reinforced by some experimental research of some twenty-five years ago. Two psychologists then tested a random sample of 115 children referred to a clinic for the treatment of dyslexia (word blindness). Of these, 112 (97 percent) showed evidence of cerebellar-vestibular dysfunction—that is, in balancing and judging distance.[17] One of the main motor functions of the cerebellum is the control of balance and other fine movement. Dyslexic children have been shown to exhibit defects in these abilities. Here, then, is a strong link between cerebellar malfunction and difficulty with reading and writing—abilities normally considered to be functions of cognition, and exclusively under cerebral (not cerebellar) control.

    (We recall that Sandy, the witch of our first chapter, suffered from dyslexia and also that she was left-handed.)

13. One of the functions of the cerebellum is the control of balance—and we refer to a mentally ill individual as "unbalanced."

14. James Prescott is another American neuropsychologist who has specialized in the study of the cerebellum. He has shown that baby apes reared in the absence of their mothers not only evidenced considerable damage to the inter-cell connections of the cerebrum, which had been known for some time, but that these deprived infants show more massive damage still to the structure of the cerebellum. While some of this cerebellar damage must be purely motor—since the deprived infant spends much of its time not moving—Prescott argues that much of it must also be due to emotional deprivation and that the socially and sexually extremely deviant behaviors of such a deprived ape when fully grown are due to cerebellar malfunction and not to cerebral malfunction. Here, then, we seem to have still further evidence of the direct role of the cerebellum in the adult's social and sexual personality.[18]

15. From several points of view the cerebellum is not simply the second most highly evolved organ this planet has ever produced, but *the* most highly evolved. The Purkinje cells of the cerebellum, for example, can each form as many as 100,000 connections with other fiber bodies—whereas a more usual figure for the cells of the cerebrum is 1,000 connections per cell. In addition, there are more cells in the granular layer of the cerebellar cortex alone *than in the whole of the rest of the brain put together.* Prescott comments dryly: "It would appear that such cell density would involve more than the regulation of motor functions."

16. The cerebellum receives "massive input" from every part of the frontal lobes of the cerebrum. These frontal areas of our brain are among the so-called silent areas of the cerebrum: that is to say, their functions are not yet understood—but it is commonly hypothesized that the frontal areas are involved in our most complex and most recently evolved thought processes. What, then, is the significance of the close relationship of these frontal areas with the cerebellum?

17. Reverting to the evolutionary history of the cerebellum, astonishingly, this organ did once, in our pre-mammalian past, possess its

own eyes. The additional pair of eyes was located on top of the head. In the course of further evolution, these eyes sank down into the brain, fused together, and became our pineal gland. Can there be any possible association between this former pair of eyes, now a single gland, and the staring single eye perceived in some before demonic manifestations (see chapter 1)? The ancient Hindus, at any rate, referred to the pineal gland as "the third eye," and as such it is known to present-day mysticism.

The foregoing points together constitute a striking prima facie case for the cerebellum as the seat of an alternative consciousness. It is a brain within the brain, a complete organism within the organism. Not only does it have informational access to all sensory and motor systems, but full executive control if the situation so merits. That full executive control, overriding any current conscious decisions or wishes, is frequently exercised in states of fear, panic, anger, sexual arousal, deprivation, and exhaustion—in short, in all kinds of emergency and extreme conditions. Why, in principle, should not the cerebellum exercise such control on other occasions also?

Despite the considerable powers of autonomy of the cerebellum, we must nevertheless appreciate that its relationship with the cerebrum is that of Siamese twin. In the final analysis the two are inseparably joined—and in this context we can probably understand, psychologically and physiologically, the clinging figure of the Old Man of the Sea. As with true Siamese twins, the attempt to separate the two physically or finally results in the effective death of both. If the cerebral cortex of a person is destroyed in an accident, or when it is experimentally destroyed in an animal, we are left with a still-living organism that is little better than a vegetable. Nevertheless, both the decerebrate human and animal continue to manifest the normal cycle of dreams, as evidenced by rapid eye movements, twitches of the face and limbs, and so on.[19] What is taking place in the residual consciousness of the organism we cannot tell—whether, in fact, the visual representation of dreams is occurring, or not. Perhaps the cerebrum is necessary for the images of dreaming to occur.

That is a matter for debate. But in the continuation of at least the physiological signs of dreaming in the decerebrate human and animal, we have clear evidence that the cerebellum and the lower brain centers *are* the physical base of dreams.

The purely physical position of the cerebellum in relation to the cerebrum accounts very well for the widespread instinctive feeling throughout mankind that the unconscious is somehow "below," and for the idea that demons lurk *behind* on the lonely road, or that if you stare in a mirror long enough, the devil will peer over your shoulder.

Incubi, succubi, demons, and poltergeists are not, after all, visitations from another world. No less amazingly, they seem to be visitations from another brain; we are haunted, it seems, by aspects of ourselves.

18
C⊕NCLUSI⊕NS

One of the clear conclusions of this survey is not simply that incubi, succubi, and poltergeists are real, but that these phenomena are aspects of the human mind, not independent supernatural entities. Such a conclusion must, nevertheless, be seen in its wider context. It then becomes clear that modern western psychology, in its total denial of these phenomena, is itself nothing more than an elaborate psychological defense mechanism against them. Modern psychology is an attempt by the conscious mind, and its chief ally science, to wholly deny the existence of its equal but opposite partner, the unconscious mind.

It is only in the past twenty-five years or so that the terms "mind" and "consciousness" have been admitted into modern academic psychology—thanks to the efforts of humanistic psychologists like Abraham Maslow and humanistic psychiatrists like R. D. Laing. The extremely influential movement, behaviorism, had dispensed with such concepts altogether, claiming that all that was needed was to observe the expressed behavior of organisms in order to understand them totally. (Yet probably this step of denying even such actually self-evident matters as mind and consciousness is only really a strategy to rule totally out of court the unconscious and the unconscious mind.) Experimental psychology in general argued much the same position as behaviorism: that there was no need to conjecture or speculate what might be going on in any organism's alleged mind. Present the organism with stimuli in a controlled situation, observe the response, and from that stimulus-response event deduce the organism's entire psychology.

Ernest Hilgard and others (chapter 7) have beautifully turned the tables on the behaviorists and the experimentalists. Precisely by controlled experiments in hypnotism they have demonstrated the existence of both mind and consciousness. In these hypnotic experiments, consciousness is divorced from mind, so that mind can conduct conversations with the hypnotist (through automatic writing) or perform mental arithmetic, or write letters to friends, while consciousness does something else. In other cases, consciousness can observe and comment upon these independent activities of mind. As for the truly unconscious mind, both hypnotic regression and deep automatic writing demonstrate its existence beyond any dispute. These are all experimental situations.

The problems facing the design of an adequate human psychology, as well as the explanation of the events described in this book, are precisely those of mind and consciousness. There is, on the one hand, no dispute about the basic two-compartment arrangement of a conscious mind allied to an unconscious mind, although the problems of exactly how the two interrelate are formidable. A more major difficulty, however, is whether we possess one consciousness, or two. Is the unconscious, perhaps, an evolved mind without its own consciousness?

Nevertheless, arguments can be made out for our possessing two different kinds of consciousness, one produced by the (so-called) conscious mind and another by the (so-called) unconscious mind. On this view, the first form, waking consciousness, is operative by day, and the second form, "sleeping" or "alternative" consciousness, is operative by night, notably during dreams. At night what we call waking consciousness is then itself unconscious, just as by day the suggested "alternative" consciousness is in turn unconscious. This description of events, in conventional language, is a little clumsy, by reason of the prejudice inherent in the terms conscious and unconscious. Who after all *says* that the unconscious is not conscious—why, waking consciousness of course! We can only describe the possible position without prejudice and without the question-begging terms of our language, by speaking of consciousness A and consciousness B. When consciousness A is switched on, consciousness B is switched off, and vice versa.

There is a case, then, for such a view of two forms of alternating consciousness, and this was presented in detail in an earlier book, *Total Man*.[1] Every individual, however, is in a position to form some kind of judgment of his or her own. The question to ask yourself is: am I the same person—am I the same me—when I am dreaming as when I am awake? It is not a question that is all that easy to answer.

Nevertheless, a rather better case can be made out for our possessing *one* form of consciousness only *that moves between the two minds* (the conscious and the unconscious), taking on the characteristics of each respective mind as it does so (see again *Total Man*). For it is perhaps the case that pure consciousness possesses no attributes of its own whatsoever, apart from self awareness. All its other apparent attributes may be derived from mind, that is, from the fact that consciousness extends itself into mind, so causing aspects of mind to become, temporarily, conscious.

If all this sounds a little wild, let us consider memory, an aspect of mind. We can summon up events from memory at will, but until we do they are not in our consciousness. They were not conscious before we summoned them up, nor are they when we let them go again. Clearly, they possess no consciousness of their own: but they can be *made* conscious. And then, what of temporary forgetting? We know that the name we want is in our head somewhere—but for the moment we cannot find it. It is out of consciousness, even though it is still in mind. Even "permanently" forgotten material, such as events from early childhood, can be recovered under hypnosis, as demonstrated in several earlier chapters. Under hypnosis this material is once again invested with consciousness (which may possibly be consciousness B)—often only temporarily, however. Roused from hypnotic trance, the individual concerned may once more be unable to recall the material.

The notion of consciousness as a naked piece of self-awareness that clothes itself in the attributes it finds in the mind[2] is a particularly useful one when we come to consider the paranormal and alternative phenomena described throughout this book. Briefly, is it the case that the naked consciousness that can cross from the conscious mind fully over into the unconscious mind then becomes the magician and the sorcerer?

Matters are a little complicated, however. For instance, when a succubus or a poltergeist visits me (from the unconscious mind) I perceive it from my position of normal consciousness in the conscious mind (so that it may make me afraid). What exactly is transpiring here?

The position appears to be that the conscious mind can perceive and become aware of the unconscious mind, and vice versa. Each mind can see the other as a set of external events. Ghosts, incubi, poltergeists, past lives, and so on are examples of the unconscious mind being seen or experienced by the conscious mind. Examples of the conscious mind being perceived by the unconscious mind—which we find in dreams, fairy stories, legends, and other products of the unconscious—are the sun and the sun-god, King Midas, the knight in shining armor, daylight itself (consider how the vampire is destroyed by daylight), the breaking of the spell (and specifically the breaking of the mirror, that destroys the mirror image, which is the alternative universe), requests for material pledges (here we think of the fairy gold that turns to dross back in the real world) or proof of identity (as when we demand the magical person's name; the unconscious mind has no permanent identity, as the conscious mind understands it), and so on. Much more information on these points has already been given in earlier books.[3]

The unconscious mind completely ceases to be frightening once we truly recognize and accept it as an integral part of ourselves, and more particularly, once we have made ourselves truly *of* it. Dreaming, as experienced by most people, is not a sufficient baptism into the unconscious mind. Something more than that is required. Nevertheless, the fact that every individual, however negative and dismissive, dreams every night is evidence for the absolute refusal of mental life to be reduced to mere waking consciousness, and at the same time confirmation of our birthright: not one universe, but two.

Consciousness possesses those powers of mind that the particular mind in question is able to confer upon it. Logical thought, objective analysis, mathematics, physics, and all the sciences are the gifts of the conscious mind to the consciousness inhabiting it.

The gifts that the unconscious mind confers upon consciousness, the more so the more completely we enter it, are artistic creativity, telepathy, clairvoyance, precognition, increased powers of self-healing and other-healing,[4] and direct access to a universe of inner beauty, which I attempted to describe in chapter 16. These do not exhaust the possibilities. As we have seen, there remain persistent claims that our other mind may be able to cause matter to travel paranormally over distance—also through solid objects in its path—and perhaps even through time,[5] and that thought forms or ideas may take on some kind of objective existence. The extreme form of the incubus and succubus may be compounded of (a) a hypnotic self-illusion plus (b) a collective hallucination involving other people plus (c) a poltergeist ability to move objects. These three items taken together *could* account for Carlotta Moran's experience in chapter 2. Or it may be that the thought form turns into some kind of real and independent entity, with some kind of objective, physical existence, as, for instance, Tibetan and other mystics have long maintained. (As said earlier, Carlos Castaneda has written extensively of these matters in his Don Juan books.)

The conscious mind works by taking in information through the senses, and so produces an internal representation of external events. In this sense, the stars and the mountains are in our heads. Since the unconscious mind works diametrically oppositely to the conscious mind, may it be that its ultimate destiny, its ultimate power, is *to produce external representations of that which it creates internally*—in the first instance as hallucinations, but in the final stage as real, solid objects?

Whether or not all this speculation concerning the unconscious mind is correct, one emphatic point is that you cannot "take it or leave it." You cannot adopt the position that you do not care whether you have an unconscious mind or not—not simply because you actually have, but because its neglect or abuse leads to very serious consequences.

In chapter 17, I suggested that nature initially set out to make the cerebellum the headquarters of the entire nervous system, but then "changed its mind" and developed the cerebrum instead. Actually, that statement is not quite true: the cerebrum was not so much developed instead of but as well as the cerebellum. In the period in which the cerebrum came to prominence, for example, the cerebellum more than doubled its own size. There were, however, losses. As we have seen, the two eyes that the cerebellum once possessed, fused together and sank down into the brain to become the single organ, the pineal gland. At the same time there were gains. With the evolution of the mammals, the cerebellum developed its own sensory pathways quite separate from those of the cerebrum. It became also undisputed controller of the autonomic nervous system.

The crucial point, possibly, is that at the same time as the cerebellum achieved independence, dreaming first appears in mammals. (Equally, as we have seen, experimental electrical stimulation of the cerebellum in the laboratory produces the physiological reactions observed during dreaming.) Is it the case that the evolved and independent cerebellum demands its own "broadcasting time," its own chance to live as nature once intended? Are dreams the broadcasting time demanded and actually achieved by the cerebellum?

The position appears to be that within each of us, sharing the protection of the same skull, lives another being with another brain—a Hyde within our Jekyll, a hunchback in our personal Notre Dame. Some kind of intuitive appreciation of this position appears to lie behind our fascination with tales of the kind just mentioned (especially with the vampire) with the ventriloquist and his dummy, with our mirror image, and much, much else of a similar nature.[6]

More to the point for the present book, however, is what happens when we do not give Hyde (or the devil) his due. What happens when we try to live as if we were just cerebral, controlled, unemotional, predictable, conscious beings—in other words when we try to live wholly in the context of the modern atheistic Western world? The answer appears to be that the unconscious steps in to take by force (or perhaps by gradual attrition) its withheld portion.

In a reasonably integrated or balanced individual (interestingly, a balance means a pivot bearing *two* equal weights), the two minds, conscious and unconscious, live together in reasonable harmony. Night dreams are vivid and intriguing, perhaps once in a while precognitive or telepathic, and often discussed. By day the unconscious is content to bubble occasional creative or fantastic or lustful thoughts through to the major partner, waking consciousness. This individual we are discussing will occasionally enjoy science fiction or fantasy films, or plays concerning the occult, and reading the odd ghost story. He fully enjoys his sensual as well as his sensory being—food, sex, and so on.

The above scenario is not intended as any kind of joke. We have seen many times in the present book what happens to the individual whose fantasy and sexual life is curtailed and repressed in childhood. We observe massive and often permanent breakdown of the adult personality. But given even the modest outlets just described, the unconscious will stockpile for ever its endless characters, its nonstop novels, its free trips to wonderland, its very evolutionary destiny, without complaint.

Speaking impressionistically, what appears to happen in the illness known as neurosis is that the conscious mind seems to become the slave of the unconscious mind. Instead of behaving in its own typical way— logically, rationally, neutrally, coherently—the conscious mind becomes irrational and emotional, beset with illogical fears of all kinds. In psychosis and schizophrenia the position is still more extreme. It is as if the conscious mind had been totally invaded and permanently taken over by the unconscious. The barrier (a permeable barrier, nevertheless) that normally operates between the conscious and the unconscious minds seems to have been entirely dismantled and destroyed. Still speaking in this impressionistic way, the extreme form of neurosis known as multiple personality appears to be a midway condition between enslavement and total invasion. Stopping short of actual invasion, the unconscious mind nevertheless sets up one or more puppet rulers in the conscious mind, which take over from time to time, and which are entirely dedicated to the wishes and policies of the unconscious (e.g., to permitting the full acting out of the latent, denied and repressed sexuality of the individual concerned).

This suggestion of neurosis and psychosis being the consequence of a battle between the conscious and unconscious minds does not at all conflict with the probability that psychosis has some structural or organic component, or with recent research that suggests that schizophrenia is the result of a viral infection.[7] The case that mind, and attributes or states of mind, are heavily involved in all illness—from the common cold (which happens to be a virus) to cancer—is, thank heavens, one that medical science today accepts. Why, then, should it be any less likely that an attitude of mind (particularly a strong conscious rejection or denial of legitimate unconscious wishes and needs) should predispose an individual to the viral infection of schizophrenia?

We know also (see chapter 13) that women are more predisposed to develop neurosis, and men more predisposed to psychosis. We know too that women have larger cerebella than men, and that women hypnotize more easily than men, i.e., are less resistant to the unconscious than men. The greater resistance of the male conscious mind to unconscious influences perhaps ultimately produces a more severe breakdown when the two minds move into conflict.

Probably the greatest stumbling block to the views of academic psychologists and psychiatrists who wish to regard all mental illness as the by-product or symptom of organic, physiological disorder—and so effectively ignore all question of powers of mind or consciousness—is the fact that mediums and psychics can turn on many of the symptoms of psychosis and neurosis at will, and equally quickly turn them off again! Thus the medium hears disembodied voices and sees visions, just like any schizophrenic or extreme neurotic. They really do hear and see them, as I can personally vouch for as a former medium. They also go into trance, and are taken over by other fully fledged personalities, just like the sufferer from multiple personality. Again, there is no playacting here: the takeover is real enough. So, if neurosis and psychosis are produced solely by chemical and hormonal imbalances, by structural defects and brain damage, how does the psychic manage to create and uncreate such imbalance and damage at the snap of the fingers?

Few would seriously dispute, of course, that the physical brain in some sense produces the mind and consciousness. A recent case, for instance, has demonstrated that total amnesia due to nerve damage can be completely and instantly cured by the introduction, in chemical form, of a single modified brain hormone.[8] Acceptance of the relationship of physical and mental life is quite a different matter, however, from agreeing that brain and mind (and consciousness) are the same commodity. On the contrary, there is now growing experimental evidence that mind is a "field" generated by the brain, and that within that field mental events organize themselves on a basis that is by no means wholly dictated by the physical brain. For example, Paul Pietsch, working with salamanders, has shown that if the two cerebral hemispheres of an adult animal are surgically removed and replaced in opposite positions, the behavior of the animal, once it recovers from surgery, is totally unaffected.[9] Again, the recent development of the brain scanner has led to the discovery of a number of outwardly normal human beings (one of whom has an IQ of 126 and a first-class honors degree in mathematics) who as a result of childhood illness have heads largely filled with cerebrospinal fluid.[10] In one case the cerebral cortex was 1 millimeter in thickness as opposed to the normal 4½ *centimeters.* Another had a brain that was "the size of a walnut." Quite clearly, then, mind and brain tissue are two very different commodities.

The weight of evidence in this book is that the many kinds of phenomena described and instanced are by far best understood as aspects of human mind, having a human causation and a human explanation. There is very little evidence for any otherworldly or afterlife origin for these phenomena, even for mediumistic phenomena. What we need as a minimum, in order to favor an extraterrestrial or afterlife source for the alleged spirits contacted by mediums and their communications, is extensive "hard" or scientific information not known to any living human being. This is what we never get. There is too a tremendous overlap in all the various forms of phenomena, and the person who produces one may very well produce others. Thus Matthew Manning, for example, produces poltergeist phenomena, automatic writing, telepathy, and psychic healing. Ruth, who suffered from multiple personality, is also telepathic. Mediumistic automatic writing can also be produced by hitherto unremarkable individuals under hypnosis, as can past-life regressions, which strikingly remind us both of true mediumistic trance and the condition of multiple personality.

In summary, then, the proposal is that all the phenomena described in this book be regarded as aspects of each other, and not as separate manifestations, as hitherto the practice in paranormal studies. All seem to be manifestations of the unconscious mind.

Therefore, far from supporting the religious view of these various matters, the recommendation here is that they should be removed from the hands of religion altogether. Just as Ufologists, with their misguided belief that unidentified objects seen in the sky are vehicles from outer space, prevent any real understanding of the phenomena concerned, so religionists through the ages have assigned the matters under discussion to the activities of spirits, demons, devils, gods, angels, and ghosts. This total error has effectively prevented any useful or meaningful investigation of the area in question.

Here in conclusion is just one more example of how religion traditionally handles these matters. The writer is a Franciscan theologian.

Sometimes, it is true, women have been seen in the woods, in the fields, in groves and dingles, lying on their backs, naked to their very navels in the posture of venery, all their limbs quivering with the orgiastic spasm. . . . In such a case there would be a very strong suspicion of the crime of demoniality, particularly if supported by other signs; and I am inclined to believe that such a circumstance, sufficiently proved by good witnesses, would justify the Judge in resorting to torture in order to ascertain the truth. . . .[11]

So much, too, for the kindly reputation of the Franciscans.

19

THE FIRST
SENSIBLE RESEARCH
PROGRAM

In Arthur C. Clarke's novel *Childhood's End,* visitors from outer space search earth's libraries to establish how far humanity has progressed with research into the paranormal. It is the only aspect of our culture that interests them. Science, they suggest—in which they are vastly superior to us—is a blind alley as far as evolutionary development is concerned, and such proves to be the case in the novel's denouement.[1]

There is much that intuitively appeals in Arthur Clarke's story, but it is, of course, fiction. However, let us suppose that real visitors from outer space appear and make a detailed inquiry into our handling of the paranormal issue. All members of the outer space committee would certainly endorse the report's undoubted main conclusion, that research into the paranormal on earth had been handled not only with a minute fraction of the funds and effort that the subject merited, but with total incompetence (or at very best with total lack of imagination) on the part of all concerned. Two of the specific criticisms of the committee would certainly be these: that despite the strongest indications of the importance of the left in the occult traditions of every culture on earth, no attempt whatsoever was made to test the psychic potential of left-handed individuals compared with that of right-handers. Similarly, despite the strongest indications from all cultures of the association of the "female principle" with the occult, no attempt was made to test the psychic potential of women against that of men. An equally obvious approach, the committee notes, would have been to test the psychic abilities of children against those of adults.

The vast majority of experimental tests on individuals conducted by the various societies for psychical research have, in any case, been basically misconceived. Always the approach has been to compare the scores obtained against the values we would expect to arise by chance. Chance situations operate as follows. If I hide a pea under one of five walnut shells and ask you to guess which shell covers the pea, chance expects you to guess correctly on average once in every five attempts. (With six shells you would be right by chance once in every six guesses, and so on.) If, however, over a large number of trials, you were scoring at an average rate of two correct out of five, or even one and a half correct out of five, the experimenter, to explain the production of such above-chance scores, would have to conclude that you were drawing on some form of paranormal guessing ability.

One of the great weaknesses of this approach of comparing actual scores achieved with the score expected by chance is that, supposing you actually paranormally perceived the hidden pea once in a hundred attempts, in addition to your correct chance guesses, that fact would not show up statistically. It would be completely lost in the flow of chance events.

In fact, the statistical concept of chance is of very little use in studying any type of human psychological affairs, let alone the paranormal. To take one example, if a man who had told the truth all his life on one occasion told a lie, that event would be totally nonexistent statistically. Statistically there is no difference between one out of a million and zero out of a million. Yet in *human* terms that single lie would be of the greatest interest. What set of circumstances, we would inquire eagerly, could have led this otherwise honorable man to break the code of a lifetime? A more appropriate example for our subject matter is as follows. Suppose in a whole lifetime of dreams a person had one single clairvoyant or telepathic dream. It might be on the occasion of the death of an absent dear friend or relative. Perhaps in the dream you see your friend lying dead. In the context of a couple of million dreams (in the course of, say, a sixty-year life) that event is statistically a complete non-event—even if you did dream it on the night of the death of that person.

We must, therefore, totally abandon in paranormal research the practice of testing scores, or other events, against chance expectations. Instead, in the testing situation, we should compare the achievements of individuals only against those of other individuals, the scores of groups only against those of other groups. Thus, if we compare the scores of a thousand men against those of a thousand women (and, ultimately, those of a hundred thousand men against those of a hundred thousand women), any slight difference that may exist between the sexes becomes additive. If women are indeed more psychic than men, their average score will gradually creep ahead of that of the men—by how much is fairly immaterial. All we need is a persistent trend in the results, however small initially. Once we have that, then we have proved the existence of the paranormal beyond any possible doubt.

This is the kind of large-scale research that must now be undertaken. Part of the beauty of the approach is that we can test a small group one day, another next week, another in a year's time, and simply add all scores together; and we can take results from Germany, America, Africa and add them on too. It does not matter where, or when, or with how many people on each occasion the test is conducted. We can even test people one at a time. They could simply drop into a bureau on the way to work, or during the lunch hour. It would not even matter if the same person took the test fifty times. No *normal* factor at all, as all scientists would agree, can produce anything but chance results in the long run. At the end of the day the average scores of both men and women ought to be absolutely identical. But if they are not, as said, we have our proof of a paranormal factor. Let us look forward to the day when we have tested twenty million women against twenty million men.

As to the tests themselves, an entire chapter would need to be written on that aspect alone. What can be said here is that the standard tests in existence—usually employing the well-known Zener cards, where subjects monotonously try to guess which of five symbols is being projected over and over again—are worse than useless. They are not productive, but destructive, of phenomena. (The Zener cards were designed with only one thought in mind—the ease with which the test results could be analyzed statistically, with never a thought for the boredom these cards generate.) What we need are standardized tests that nevertheless generate emotion and excitement. For some people, for instance, guessing against a roulette wheel when money is at stake sets the adrenaline flowing in no uncertain fashion. It requires very little imagination to devise a range of such exciting tests, but even that minute quantity of imagination seems unavailable to psychic researchers.

In any case, too much emphasis must not be placed on tests. They have their uses, even though the scientific establishment for whose benefit they are usually conducted totally ignores them, as Brian Inglis has recently stressed.[2] (However, they will not be able to ignore the cumulative scores of hundreds of thousands of men and women.) Thus the strong results obtained in controlled tests by Dr. Bernard Grad,[3] Dr. Norman Shealy,[4] and the several distinguished scientists who worked with Matthew Manning[5] were not reported or discussed in the scientific press.

Active search must also be made for the gifted psychic who can produce the really dramatic phenomena. Many of these individuals do not even realize they are psychic (as Martyn Pryer and Mrs. W. D. did not until middle life). So far in psychical research the practice has been to test any individuals available at random. This is like pulling in a hundred people off the street and expecting to find a Lester Piggott, a Fred Astaire, and an Einstein among them.

The main thrust of current laboratory research should be twofold. One, to develop techniques to improve and develop the paranormal abilities of those showing strong natural gifts. Second, to identify the precise physiological basis of paranormal abilities. Both of these approaches, but especially the latter, would again outflank the resistance of the scientific establishment. C. Maxwell Cade is pioneering the use of biofeedback equipment in the first area,[6] and many other possibilities exist, including the Christos technique[7] and the use of dream tapes.[8] The Christos technique induces experiences similar to those described at the end of chapter 16, and dream tapes encourage lucid dreaming—wherein one achieves normal consciousness without interrupting the dream. (Incidentally, dreaming is probably the very best initial road into the paranormal universe. Developing one's dreams, even by simply keeping a dream journal, a record written on waking of one's dreams of the previous night, is an excellent way to begin the development of psychic faculties. Automatic writing is another.[9])

Research in the second area, the physiological basis of paranormal abilities, should probably concentrate on the cerebellum (see chapter 17) and the autonomic nervous system generally. It is likely that psychic individuals have larger than normal cerebella, and a simple first step toward proving that this organ is indeed the seat of psychic activity would be to compare the test scores of those possessing relatively large cerebella with those possessing relatively small cerebella.

A further line of inquiry is as follows. It is very probable that our species is the outcome of the genetic crossing of two very different early varieties of man, Cro-Magnon and Neanderthal.[10] Cro-Magnon man was tall (average male height 6 feet, average female height 5 feet 6 inches) with a small cerebellum. Neanderthal was short (5 feet 4 inches average for men, 4 feet 10 inches for women) with a large cerebellum. Neanderthal was extremely mystical, as we know from the examination of Neanderthal shrines and burials. He may also have been predominantly left-handed, while Cro-Magnon was probably largely or entirely right-handed. One further anatomical feature can also be mentioned—in Neanderthal the big toe was noticeably shorter than the second toe, whereas in Cro-Magnon (as in most people today) the big toe was longer than all others (see figures 1–6).

Here, then, is a wealth of research possibilities. Do short people have larger cerebella than tall people—and so are short people more psychic than tall people? Do professional mediums tend to be of below average height? Does the possession of several of the characteristics of Neanderthal make an individual more likely to be psychic—i.e., if you are short, left-handed, with a large cerebellum and a short big toe?

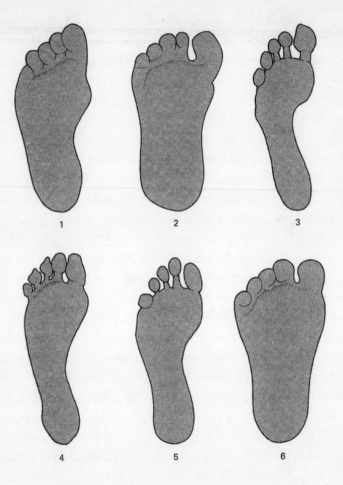

1 *Cro-Magnon man (footprint in clay, around 25,000 years old)*
2 *Neanderthal man (footprint in clay, at least 35,000 years old)*
3 *Typical modern European foot*
4 *Footprint of Mr. W. G., a living, left-handed white adult male*
5 *Footprint of Mrs. C. W., a living, left-handed white female*
6 *Footprint of the legendary Yeti or Bigfoot (sketch of track in mud, Russia)*

We have commented more than once on the witch marks for which the Inquisitors searched their victims—namely, extra nipples and large warts. Is it possible that Neanderthal man tended to have supernumerary nipples, and a tendency to produce warts? The idea is not totally absurd. Sandy, in chapter 1, has an extra nipple and is left-handed. Mr. W. G., whose foot with its short big toe is shown in figure 4, is also left-handed, is 5 feet 5 inches tall, has a large head in relation to his body (a known Neanderthal characteristic)—and warts. He also experiences lucid dreams. Mrs. C. W. also has the short big toe (see figure 5), is left-handed, has no earlobes (a possible Neanderthal characteristic), and is 5 feet 2 inches tall—"the tallest female in her family." A recent reference book (*Growth,* Time-Life International, 1966) proposes an average height of 5 feet 9 inches for British adult males today and an average of 5 feet 4 inches for British adult females. Clearly, our two short-big-toe subjects are below present-day average height for their respective sexes.

Whether Mr. W. G., Mrs. C. W., and Sandy have large cerebella (another known Neanderthal characteristic) is a matter that would require a brain scanner to determine.

What is needed as an absolute urgency is a large research institute, preferably staffed by psychics who also have sound academic qualifications. Apart from conducting research along the kind of lines suggested, they would also be seeking to develop greater psychic abilities in young people who already show promise. The kind of phenomena that could be produced have of course already been described in detail in this book. The Philip experiment described in chapter 3 provides an excellent example to build upon. Such an institute would in the long run generate the kinds of proofs that the scientific community demands, without always following the strict scientific method that is so destructive of phenomena. As C. Brookes-Smith and D. W. Hunt remark in connection with their own production of poltergeist phenomena (chapter 3):

These experimental researches in psychokinesis were intentionally devoid of conventional control measures and there was no attempt to *prove* the reality of the observed phenomena. There was therefore complete freedom from the "crucial test" situation that leads to the most acute form of "deadly doubt" and the consequent total inhibition of phenomena. This policy has been strongly advocated by Batcheldor and was the only way to by-pass the inhibition barrier that has hampered research in this field for so long.[11]

Acupuncture and hypnosis were once dismissed by science as nonsense. These achieved recognition by the sheer scope and scale of their development—in other words, they became commonplace. Science had no option at this point but to bow to the inevitable. The paranormal, too, must become commonplace.

We cannot do better than end with a quotation from Herbert Spencer. It tells us why the many creatures from our inner space, with their altogether remarkable powers, remain unacknowledged by science: "There is a principle which is bar against all information, which is proof against all arguments, which cannot fail to keep a man in everlasting ignorance: that principle is contempt, prior to investigation."

NOTES

CHAPTER 1: INCUBI AND SUCCUBI IN SUBURBIA

1. Krishna, *Kundalini: the Evolutionary Energy in Man.*

CHAPTER 2: DEMONS PAST AND ENTITIES PRESENT

1. Jackson, *The New Schaff-Herzog Encyclopaedia of Religious Knowledge;* MacCulloch, *The Mythology of All Races;* Alexander, *The Mythology of All Races.*
2. Gooch, *The Neanderthal Question;* Shackley, *Wild Men: Yeti, Sasquatch and the Neanderthal Enigma.*
3. MacCulloch, *The Mythology of All Races;* Alexander, *The Mythology of All Races.*
4. Freud, *The Interpretation of Dreams, Standard Works,* vol. 4.; Freud, *Introductory Lectures on Psychoanalysis, Standard Works,* vols. 15 and 16.
5. Gooch, *Total Man;* Penelope Shuttle and Peter Redgrove, *The Wise Wound.*
6. *Oxford English Dictionary* (Oxford: Clarendon Press, 1933).
7. Summers, *The History of Witchcraft and Demonology.*
8. MacCulloch, *The Mythology of All Races;* Alexander, *The Mythology of All Races.*
9. Ibid.

10. Willoughby-Meade, *Chinese Ghouls and Goblins.*
11. Gooch, *The Secret Life of Humans.*
12. L'Estrange Ewen, *Witchcraft and Demonaism.*
13. Summers, *The History of Witchcraft and Demonology.*
14. Summers, *Demonality or Incubi and Succubi.*
15. Ibid.
16. De Felitta, *The Entity.*
17. Ibid.

CHAPTER 3: POLTERGEIST

1. Owen, *Can We Explain the Poltergeist?*
2. Ibid.
3. Ibid.
4. Manning, *The Link.*
5. Roll, *The Poltergeist.*
6. Ibid.
7. Ibid.
8. Manning, *The Link.*
9. Manning, *In the Minds of Millions.*
10. Durbin, "A Narrative of Some Extraordinary Things that Happened to Mr Richard Gile's Children," quoted in Owen, *Can We Explain the Poltergeist?*
11. Ibid.
12. Ibid.
13. Nielsson, *Congrès International tenu á Varsovie en 1923,* quoted in Owen, *Can We Explain the Poltergeist?*
14. Ibid.
15. Owen, *Can We Explain the Poltergeist?*
16. Ibid.
17. Ibid.
18. Roll, *The Poltergeist.*
19. Williams, "The Poltergeist Man."
20. Ibid.
21. Ibid.
22. "Philip the Man-made Phantom."
23. Prescott, "Early Somatosensory Deprivation as an Ontogenetic Process in the Abnormal Development of the Brain and Behaviour."

24. Batcheldor, "Report on a Case of Table Levitation and Associated Phenomena."
25. Ibid.
26. Brookes-Smith and Hunt, "Some Experiments in Psychokinesis."
27. Ibid.

CHAPTER 4: PARANORMAL FIRE

1. Harrison, *Fire From Heaven.*
2. Hitching, *The World Atlas of Mysteries.*
3. Harrison, *Fire From Heaven.*
4. Hitching, *The World Atlas of Mysteries.*
5. Thurston, "Preternatural Combustion of the Human Body."
6. Harrison, *Fire From Heaven.*
7. Ibid.
8. Thurston, "Preternatural Combustion of the Human Body."
9. Schurmacher, *Strange Unsolved Mysteries,* cited in Colin Wilson, *The Occult.*
10. Hitching, *The World Atlas of Mysteries.*
11. Harrison, *Fire From Heaven.*
12. Owen, *Can We Explain the Poltergeist?*
13. Harrison, *Fire From Heaven.*
14. Ibid.
15. Owen, *Can We Explain the Poltergeist?*
16. Harrison, *Fire From Heaven.*
17. Ibid.
18. Ibid.
19. Manning, *The Link.*
20. Ibid.
21. Singer, *The Seance.*

CHAPTER 5: AUTOMATIC WRITING

1. Hilgard, *Divided Consciousness: Multiple Controls in Human Thought and Action.*
2. Mühl, *Automatic Writing.*
3. Myers, "Automatic Writing III."

4. Mühl, *Automatic Writing.*
5. Messerschmidt, "A Quantitive Investigation of the Alleged Independent Operation of Conscious and Subconscious Processes."
6. James, "Automatic Writing."
7. Hilgard, *Divided Consciousness.*
8. Manning, *The Link.*
9. "New Music from Old Masters."
10. Manning, *The Strangers;* Manning, *The Link.*
11. Ibid.
12. Ibid.
13. Jenkins, *The Shadow and the Light.*

CHAPTER 6: PAST LIVES?

1. Guirdham, *We Are One Another;* Guirdham, *The Cathars and Reincarnation;* Gur, "Imagery, Absorption and the Tendency towards 'Mind Exploration' as Correlates of Hypnosis Susceptibility in Males and Females."
2. Wilson, *Mind Out Of Time?*
3. Ibid.
4. Iverson, *More Lives than One?*
5. Wilson, *Mind Out Of Time?*
6. Ibid.
7. Ibid.
8. Gooch, *The Paranormal.*
9. Jacobson, *Life Without Death?*
10. Stevenson, *Twenty Cases Suggestive of Reincarnation.*
11. Wilson, *Mind Out Of Time?*
12. Ibid.
13. Gooch, *The Paranormal.*
14. Freda Sklair, personal communication to the author.
15. Clements, "What a Fetus Hears an Adult Remembers."
16. Wilson, *Mind Out of Time?*
17. Sidis and Goodhart, *Multiple Personality.*
18. Ibid.
19. Ibid.

CHAPTER 7: HYPNOSIS

1. Hilgard, *Divided Consciousness: Multiple Controls in Human Thought and Action.*
2. Mason, "A Case of Congenital Ichthyosiform Erythrodermia Treated by Hypnosis."
3. Bettley, letter in *British Medical Journal* 2 (1952).
4. Gooch, *The Secret Life of Humans;* Osty, *Supernormal Faculties in Man.*
5. Hilgard, *Divided Consciousness.*
6. Ibid.
7. Bowers, "Sex and Susceptibility as Moderator Variables in the Relationship of Creativity and Hypnotic Susceptibility."
8. Gibson, *Hypnosis.*
9. Hilgard, *Hypnotic Susceptibility.*
10. Weitzenhoffer, *Hypnotism.*
11. Ibid.
12. Hull, *Hypnosis and Suggestibility.*
13. Gibson, *Hypnosis.*
14. Ibid.
15. Weitzenhoffer, *Hypnotism.*
16. Gur, "Imagery, Absorption and the Tendency towards 'Mind Exploration' as Correlates of Hypnosis Susceptibility in Males and Females."
17. Gur and Gur, "Handedness, Sex and Eyedness as Moderating Variables in the Relation between Hypnotic Susceptibility and Functional Brain Asymmetry."

CHAPTER 8: STIGMATA

1. Moody, "Bodily Changes During Abreaction."
2. Taylor, *The Natural History of the Mind.*
3. Wilson, *Mind Out Of Time?*
4. Spiegl, *The Life and Death of Therese Neumann of Konnersreuth.*
5. Lechler, *Das Rätsel von Konnersreuth im Lichte eines Neuen Falles von Stigmatisation.*

CHAPTER 9: MEDIUMSHIP

1. Twigg and Brod, *Ena Twigg, Medium.*
2. Ibid.
3. Phylos the Tibetan, *A Dweller on Two Planets.*
4. Roberts, *Psychic Politics.*
5. Ibid.
6. Kennedy, *The Constant Nymph.*
7. Broad, *Lectures on Psychical Research.*

CHAPTER 10: DISCARNATES?

1. Yeats, *Essays and Introductions.*
2. Schopenhauer, *Parerga and Paralipomena.*
3. Simon, "That Was No Lady, That's a Ghost."
4. Gurney, Myers, and Podmore, *Phantasms of the Living.*
5. Sidgwick, "Phantasms of the Living."
6. Gooch, *The Paranormal.*
7. Jenkins, *The Shadow and the Light.*
8. Schatzman, *The Story of Ruth.*
9. Green and McCreery, *Apparitions.*
10. Haynes, *The Hidden Springs.*
11. Gooch, *The Paranormal;* Tarver, letter, *New Scientist,* 24 October 1968.
12. Rose, *Living Magic.*
13. Rees, "The Hallucinations of Widowhood."
14. "Spontaneous Hallucinations of the Sane."
16. Schatzman, *The Story of Ruth.*
16. Ibid.

CHAPTER 11: LEFT-HANDEDNESS

1. Hertz, "The Pre-eminence of the Right Hand: a Study in Religious Polarity."
2. Chelhod, "A Contribution to the Problem of the Pre-eminence of the Right."
3. Gooch, *The Secret Life of Humans;* Gooch, *The Dream Culture of the Neanderthals;* Tomas, *We Are Not the First.*

4. Hertz, "The Pre-eminence of the Right Hand."
5. Teng et al., "Handedness in a Chinese Population."
6. Hertz, "The Pre-eminence of the Right Hand."
7. Ibid.
8. Granet, "Right and Left in China."
9. Hertz, "The Pre-eminence of the Right Hand."
10. Lloyd, "Right and Left in Greek Philosophy."
11. Evans-Pritchard, *Nuer Religion.*
12. Wieschoff, "Concepts of Right and Left in African Cultures."
13. Faron, "Symbolic Values and the Integration of Society among the Mapuche of Chile."
14. Needham, *Left and Right.*
15. "Human Brain," BBC TV, May/June 1982.
16. Dow and Moruzzi, *The Physiology and Pathology of the Cerebellum.*
17. Prescott, "Forebrain, Midbrain and Hindbrain Correlations."
18. Beck, "The Right-Left Division of South Indian Society."
19. Lloyd, "Right and Left in Greek Philosophy."
20. Chelhod, "A Contribution to the Problem of the Pre-eminence of the Right."
21. Ibid.
22. Hertz, "The Pre-eminence of the Right Hand."
23. Young and Knapp, "Personality Characteristics of Converted Left-Handers."
24. Tomoko Izumi, personal communication to the author.
25. Burt, *The Backward Child.*
26. Clark, *Teaching Left-Handed Children.*
27. Pringle, *11,000 Seven-Year-Olds.*
28. Gooch, *The Double Helix of the Mind;* Gooch, "Right Brain, Left Brain."
29. Burt, *The Backward Child.*
30. Peterson, "Left-Handedness: Differences Between Student Artists and Scientists."
31. Jung, *Aion, Collected Works,* vol. 9; Jung, *Psychology and Alchemy, Collected Works,* vol. 12; Jung, *Alchemical Studies, Collected Works,* vol. 13.
32. Sackeim et al., "Emotions Are Expressed More Intensely on the Left Side of the Face."
33. Teng et al., "Handedness in a Chinese Population."

34. Breuil and Lantier, *The Men of the Old Stone Age.*
35. Teng et al., "Handedness in a Chinese Population."
36. Gooch, *The Dream Culture of the Neanderthals;* Gooch, *The Neanderthal Question.*
37. Burt, *The Backward Child.*

CHAPTER 12: A SHORT NOTE ON UFOS

1. Clarke, *Report on Planet Three and Other Speculations.*
2. Miller, "Do the Media Create UFO Sightings?"
3. Ibid.
4. Fitzgerald, "Messages: the Case History of a Contactee."
5. Gooch and Evans, *Science Fiction as Religion.*
6. Puharich, *Uri.*

CHAPTER 13: THE DYNAMIC UNCONSCIOUS

1. Freud, *Introductory Lectures on Psychoanalysis, Standard Works,* vols. 15 and 16.
2. Freud, *The Interpretation of Dreams, Standard Works,* vol. 4.
3. Freud, *The Psychopathology of Everyday Life, Standard Works,* vol. 6.
4. Ibid.; Freud, *Introductory Lectures on Psychoanalysis, Standard Works,* vols. 15 and 16.
5. Horney, *Our Inner Conflicts;* Horney, *The Neurotic Personality of Our Time.*
6. Jung, *Memories, Dreams, Reflections;* Sulloway, *Freud, Biologist of the Mind.*
7. Jung, *Memories, Dreams, Reflections.*
8. Ibid.
9. Sulloway, *Freud, Biologist of the Mind.*
10. Shuttle and Redgrove, *The Wise Wound.*
11. Roth and Luton, "The Mental Health Programme in Tennessee."
12. Lemkau et al., "Mental-Hygiene Problems in an Urban District."
13. Lester, "Suicidal Behaviour, Sex and Mental Disorder."
14. Owen, *Can We Explain the Poltergeist?*

CHAPTER 14: MULTIPLE PERSONALITY

1. *Encyclopaedia Britannica*, 15th edition (1974), s.v. "Multiple Personality."
2. Wilson, *Mind Out Of Time?*
3. Thigpen and Cleckley, *The Three Faces of Eve.*
4. Ibid.
5. Prince, *The Dissociation of Personality.*
6. Ibid.
7. Wilson, *Mind Out Of Time?*
8. Schreiber, *Sybil.*
9. Hilgard, *Divided Consciousness: Multiple Controls in Human Thought and Action.*
10. Usher, "Can This Boy Be Ten Different People?"
11. Sidis and Goodhart, *Multiple Personality.*
12. Ibid.
13. Gooch, *Personality and Evolution.*
14. Sizemore and Pittillo, *Eve.*
15. Schreiber, *Sybil.*

CHAPTER 15: PSYCHOSIS, SCHIZOPHRENIA AND AUTISM

1. Woolf, *Beginning Again.*
2. Crowcroft, *The Psychotic.*
3. Dominian, *Psychiatry and the Christian.*
4. Crowcroft, *The Psychotic.*
5. Selfe, *Nadia—A Case of Extraordinary Drawing Ability in an Autistic Child.*
6. Ibid.
7. Wilson, *Mind Out Of Time?*
8. Stevenson, *Twenty Cases Suggestive of Reincarnation.*

CHAPTER 16: THE NATURAL HISTORY OF PSYCHICS

1. Lindsay, *William Blake.*
2. Raine, *Blake and the New Age.*
3. Lindsay, *William Blake.*
4. Ibid.

5. Mikhail, *W. B. Yeats: Interviews and Recollections.*
6. Ellman, *Yeats: the Man and the Masks.*
7. Ibid.
8. Ibid.
9. Twigg and Brod, *Ena Twigg, Medium.*
10. Gooch, *Total Man.*
11. Gooch, *The Double Helix of the Mind;* Gooch, *The Paranormal.*
12. Gooch, *The Paranormal.*
13. Kennedy, *The Constant Nymph.*
14. Gooch, *The Double Helix of the Mind;* Gooch, *The Paranormal.*
15. Crick and Mitchison, "The Function of Dream Sleep."
16. Gooch, *The Double Helix of the Mind;* Gooch, *Total Man.*

CHAPTER 17: BUT WHERE IN THE BRAIN IS THE UNCONSCIOUS?

1. Ornstein, *The Psychology of Consciousness.*
2. Gazzaniga, *The Bisected Brain.*
3. Krynauw, "Infantile Hemiplegia Treated by Removing One Cerebral Hemisphere"; McFie, "The Effects of Hemispherectomy on Intellectual Functioning in Cases of Infantile Hemiplegia."
4. McFie, "The Effects of Hemispherectomy on Intellectual Functioning in Cases of Infantile Hemiplegia."
5. Smith, "Speech and Other Functions after Left (Dominant) Hemispherectomy."
6. Gooch, *The Double Helix of the Mind.*
7. Krishna, *Kundalini: the Evolutionary Energy in Man.*
8. Bentov, *Stalking the Wild Pendulum.*
9. Barr, *The Human Nervous System.*
10. Morgan and Stellar, *Physiological Psychology.*
11. Ibid.
12. Prescott, "Forebrain, Midbrain and Hindbrain Correlations."
13. Breuil and Lantier, *The Men of the Old Stone Age.*
14. Teng et al., "Handedness in a Chinese Population."
15. Gooch, *The Double Helix of the Mind;* Gooch, *Total Man.*
16. "Human Brain," BBC TV, May/June 1982.

17. Dow and Moruzzi, *The Physiology and Pathology of the Cerebellum.*
18. Prescott, "Phylogenetic and Ontogenetic Aspects of Human Affectual Development"; Prescott, "Early Somatosensory Deprivation as an Ontogenetic Process in the Abnormal Development of the Brain and Behaviour."
19. Oswald, *Sleep.*

CHAPTER 18: CONCLUSIONS

1. Gooch, *Total Man.*
2. Gooch, *Personality and Evolution.*
3. Gooch, *The Double Helix of the Mind;* Gooch, *Personality and Evolution;* Gooch, *Total Man.*
4. Gooch, *The Secret Life of Humans;* Gooch, *The Double Helix of the Mind;* Gooch, *The Paranormal.*
5. Manning, *The Link;* Owen, *Can We Explain the Poltergeist?*
6. Gooch, *Total Man.*
7. "Schizophrenia: The Case for Viruses."
8. Wallace, "The Day They Gave This Man His Memory Back."
9. Pietsch, *Shufflebrain.*
10. Wright, "The No-Brain Genius May Be on its Way."
11. Summers, *Demonality or Incubi and Succubi.*

CHAPTER 19: THE FIRST SENSIBLE
RESEARCH PROGRAM

1. Clarke, *Childhood's End.*
2. Inglis, in *Light* 103, no. 1 (1983).
3. Grad, "Some Biological Effects of the Laying on of Hands"; Grad et al., "The Influence of an Unorthodox Method of Treatment on Wound Healing in Mice."
4. Gooch, *The Paranormal.*
5. Manning, *The Strangers.*
6. Cade and Coxhead, *The Awakened Mind.*
7. Glaskin, *Windows of the Mind.*

8. Gooch, *The Double Helix of the Mind*.
9. Ibid.
10. Gooch, *The Dream Culture of the Neanderthals*; Gooch, *The Neanderthal Question*.
11. Brookes-Smith and Hunt, "Some Experiments in Psychokinesis."

BIBLI⊕GRAPHY

Adler, Alfred. *Practice and Theory of Individual Psychology.* London: Routledge, 1929.

Alexander, H. B., ed. *The Mythology of All Races* (12 vols.). New York: Cooper Square, 1964.

Barr, Murray L. *The Human Nervous System.* New York: Harper & Row, 1974.

Baskin, Wade. *Dictionary of Satanism.* London: Peter Owen, 1972.

Batcheldor, K. J. "Report on a Case of Table Levitation and Associated Phenomena." *Journal of the Society for Psychical Research* 43 (1966).

Beck, Brenda E. F. "The Right-Left Division of South Indian Society." In Rodney Needham, *Left and Right.* Chicago: University of Chicago Press, 1973.

Bentov, Itzhak. *Stalking the Wild Pendulum.* London: Wildwood House, 1978.

Bettley, F. R. Letter in *British Medical Journal* 2 (1952).

Bowers, K. S. "Sex and Susceptibility as Moderator Variables in the Relationship of Creativity and Hypnotic Susceptibility." *Journal of Abnormal Psychology* 78 (1971).

Breuil, Henri, and Raymond Lantier. *The Men of the Old Stone Age.* London: Harrap, 1965.

Broad, C. D. *Lectures on Psychical Research.* London: Routledge, 1962.

Brookes-Smith, C., and D. W. Hunt. "Some Experiments in Psychokinesis." *Journal of the Society for Psychical Research* 45 (1970).

Burt, Cyril. *The Backward Child.* London: University of London, 1937.

Cade, Maxwell C., and Nona Coxhead. *The Awakened Mind.* London: Wildwood House, 1979.

Chelhod, J. "A Contribution to the Problem of the Pre-eminence of the Right." In Rodney Needham, *Left and Right.* Chicago: University of Chicago Press, 1973.

Clark, Margaret. *Teaching Left-Handed Children.* London: University of London, 1959.

Clarke, Arthur C. *Report on Planet Three and Other Speculations.* London: Corgi Books, 1975.

———. *Childhood's End.* London: Pan, 1954.

Clements, Michele. "What a Fetus Hears an Adult Remembers." *General Practitioner,* 13 April (1979).

Cooper, I. S., M. Riklan, and R. S. Snider. "The Effect of Cerebellar Lesions on Emotional Behaviour in the Rhesus Monkey." In *The Cerebellum, Epilepsy and Behaviour.* New York: Plenum Press, 1972.

Cramer, Marc. *The Devil Within.* London: W. H. Allen, 1979.

Crick, Francis, and Graeme Mitchison. "The Function of Dream Sleep." *Nature* 11 (1983).

Crowcroft, Andrew. *The Psychotic.* Harmondsworth: Penguin, 1975.

Dominian, J. *Psychiatry and the Christian.* London: Burns & Oates, 1962.

Dow, R. S., and G. Moruzzi. *The Physiology and Pathology of the Cerebellum.* Minneapolis: University of Minnesota, 1958.

Durbin, Henry. "A Narrative of Some Extraordinary Things that Happened to Mr Richard Gile's Children." (Bristol, 1800) In A. R. G. Owen, *Can We Explain the Poltergeist?* New York: Helix Press, 1964.

Ellman, Richard. *Yeats: the Man and the Masks.* Oxford: Oxford University Press, 1979.

Evans-Pritchard, E. E. *Nuer Religion.* Oxford: Oxford University Press, 1956.

L'Estrange Ewen, C. H. *Witchcraft and Demonaism.* London: Cranton, 1933.

Faron, Louis C. "Symbolic Values and the Integration of Society among the Mapuche of Chile." In Rodney Needham, *Left and Right.* Chicago: University of Chicago Press, 1973.

De Felitta, Frank. *The Entity.* London: Collins, 1979.

Fitzgerald, Randy. "Messages: the Case History of a Contactee." *Second Look,* October (1979).

Fox, James J. "On Bad Death and the Left Hand." In Rodney Needham, *Left and Right*. Chicago: University of Chicago Press, 1973.

Frankel, F. H., and H. S. Zamansky (eds.). *Hypnosis at its Bicentennial*. New York: Plenum Press, 1978.

Freud, Sigmund. *The Interpretation of Dreams, Standard Works*, vol. 4. London: Hogarth, 1958.

———. *The Psychopathology of Everyday Life, Standard Works*, vol. 6. London: Hogarth, 1960.

———. *Introductory Lectures on Psychoanalysis, Standard Works*, vols. 15 and 16. London: Hogarth, 1963.

Gardner, W. J., et al. "Residual Function Following Hemispherectomy for Tumour and Infantile Hemiplegia." *Brain* 78 (1955).

Gazzaniga, M. S. *The Bisected Brain*. New York: Meredith Corporation, 1970.

Gibson, H. B. *Hypnosis*. London: Peter Owen, 1977.

Glaskin, G. M. *Windows of the Mind*. London: Wildwood House, 1975.

Goldsmith, I. E., and J. Moor-Jankowski. *Medical Primatology*. New York: Karger, 1971.

Gooch, Stan. *The Dream Culture of the Neanderthals*. Rochester, Vt.: Inner Traditions, 2006.

———. "Left-handedness." *New Scientist*, 22 July (1982).

———. *The Secret Life of Humans*. London: Dent, 1981.

———. *The Double Helix of the Mind*. London: Wildwood House, 1980.

———. "Right Brain, Left Brain," *New Scientist*, 11 September (1980).

———. *The Paranormal*. London: Wildwood House, 1978.

———. *The Neanderthal Question*. London: Wildwood House, 1977.

———. *Personality and Evolution*. London: Wildwood House, 1973.

———. *Total Man*. London: Allen Lane, 1972.

Gooch, Stan, and Chris Evans. *Science Fiction as Religion*. Frome, Somerset: Brans Head Press, 1980.

Grad, Bernard. "Some Biological Effects of the Laying on of Hands." *Journal of the American Society for Psychical Research* 59 (1965).

Grad, Bernard, et al. "The Influence of an Unorthodox Method of Treatment on Wound Healing in Mice." *International Journal of Parapsychology* 3, no. 2 (1961).

Granet, Marcel. "Right and Left in China." In Rodney Needham, *Left and Right*. Chicago: University of Chicago Press, 1973.

Green, Celia, and Charles McCreery. *Apparitions*. London: Hamish Hamilton, 1975.

Guirdham, Arthur. *The Lake and the Castle*. London: Spearman (Jersey), 1976.

———. *We Are One Another*. London: Spearman (Jersey), 1974.

———. *The Cathars and Reincarnation*. London: Spearman (Jersey), 1970.

Gur, Ruben C. "Imagery, Absorption and the Tendency towards 'Mind Exploration' as Correlates of Hypnosis Susceptibility in Males and Females." In F. H. Frankel and H. S. Zamansky, eds., *Hypnosis at its Bicentennial*. New York: Plenum Press, 1978.

Gur, Ruben C., and Raquel E. Gur. "Handedness, Sex and Eyedness as Moderating Variables in the Relation between Hypnotic Susceptibility and Functional Brain Asymmetry." *Journal of Abnormal Psychology* 83 (1974).

Gurney, E., F. W. H. Myers, and F. Podmore. *Phantasms of the Living*, 2 vols. London: Trübner, 1886.

Harrison, Michael. *Fire From Heaven*. London: Sidgwick & Jackson, 1976.

Haynes, Renée. *The Hidden Springs*. London: Hollis & Carter, 1961.

Hertz, Robert. "The Pre-eminence of the Right Hand: a Study in Religious Polarity." In Rodney Needham, *Left and Right*. Chicago: University of Chicago Press, 1973.

Hilgard, Ernest R. *Divided Consciousness: Multiple Controls in Human Thought and Action*. New York: Wiley, 1977.

———. *Hypnotic Susceptibility*. New York: Harcourt Brace, 1968.

Hitching, Francis. *The World Atlas of Mysteries*. London: Collins, 1978.

Horney, Karen. *Our Inner Conflicts*. London: Routledge, 1946.

———. *The Neurotic Personality of Our Time*. London: Routledge, 1937.

Hull, C. L. *Hypnosis and Suggestibility*. New York: Appleton-Century, 1933.

"Human Brain." BBC TV, May/June 1982.

Inglis, Brian. In *Light* 103, no. 1 (1983).

Iverson, Jeffrey. *More Lives than One?* London: Souvenir Press, 1976.

Iyengar, B. K. S. *Light on Pranayama*. London: Allen & Unwin, 1981.

Izumi, Tomoko. Personal communication to the author.

Jackson, S. M., ed. *The New Schaff-Herzog Encyclopaedia of Religious Knowledge*. New York: Funk & Wagnall, 1909.

Jacobson, Nils. *Life Without Death?* New York: Delacorte Press, 1973.

James, William. "Automatic Writing." *Proceedings*, American Society for Psychical Research 1 (1889).

Jastrzembska, Z. S., ed. *The Effects of Blindness and Other Impairments on Early Development.* New York: American Foundation for the Blind, 1976.

Jenkins, Elizabeth. *The Shadow and the Light.* London: Hamilton, 1982.

Jung, C. G. *Memories, Dreams, Reflections.* London: Routledge, 1963.

———. *Aion, Collected Works,* vol. 9. London: Routledge, 1959

———. *Psychology and Alchemy, Collected Works,* vol. 12. London: Routledge, 1959.

———. *Alchemical Studies, Collected Works,* vol. 13. London: Routledge, 1959.

Kennedy, Margaret. *The Constant Nymph.* London: Heinemann, 1924.

Kolb, L. C. *Modern Clinical Psychiatry.* London: Saunders, 1977.

Krishna, Gopi. *Kundalini: the Evolutionary Energy in Man.* London: Stuart, 1970.

Kruyt, A. C. "Right and Left in Central Celebes." In Rodney Needham, *Left and Right.* Chicago: University of Chicago Press, 1973.

Krynauw, Rowland A. "Infantile Hemiplegia Treated by Removing One Cerebral Hemisphere." *Journal of Neurology, Neurosurgery and Psychiatry* 13 (1950).

Lechler, Alfred. *Das Rätsel von Konnersreuth im Lichte eines Neuen Falles von Stigmatisation.* Elberfeld, 1933.

Lemkau, P., et al. "Mental-Hygiene Problems in an Urban District." *Mental Hygiene* 26 (1942).

Lester, David. "Suicidal Behaviour, Sex and Mental Disorder." *Psychological Reports* 27 (1970).

———. "Suicidal Behaviour in Men and Women." *Mental Hygiene* 53 (1969).

Lindsay, Jack. *William Blake.* London: Constable, 1978.

Lloyd, Geoffrey. "Right and Left in Greek Philosophy." In Rodney Needham, *Left and Right.* Chicago: University of Chicago Press, 1973.

MacCulloch, J. A., ed. *The Mythology of All Races,* 13 vols. Boston: Marshall James, 1930.

Manning, Matthew. *The Strangers.* London: W. H. Allen, 1978.

———. *In the Minds of Millions.* London: W. H. Allen, 1977.

———. *The Link.* London: Colin Smythe, 1974.

Mason, A. A. "A Case of Congenital Ichthyosiform Erythrodermia Treated by Hypnosis." *British Medical Journal* 2 (1952).

McFie, John. "The Effects of Hemispherectomy on Intellectual Functioning in Cases of Infantile Hemiplegia." *Journal of Neurology, Neurosurgery and Psychiatry* 24 (1961).

Messerschmidt, R. "A Quantitive Investigation of the Alleged Independent Operation of Conscious and Subconscious Processes." *Journal of Abnormal and Social Psychology* 22 (1927–8).

Mikhail, E. H. *W. B. Yeats: Interviews and Recollections.* London: Macmillan, 1977.

Miller, Ron. "Do the Media Create UFO Sightings?" *Second Look,* November/December (1979).

Moody, R. L. "Bodily Changes During Abreaction." *Lancet* 251, no. 2 (1946), and vol. 254, no. 2, (1948).

Morgan, C. T., and E. Stellar. *Physiological Psychology.* New York: McGraw Hill, 1950.

Mühl, Anita. *Automatic Writing.* New York: Helix Press, 1930.

Myers, F. W. H. "Automatic Writing III." *Proceedings,* Society for Psychical Research, vol. 4 (1887).

Needham, Rodney. *Left and Right.* Chicago: University of Chicago Press, 1973.

"New Music from Old Masters." *Alpha,* July/August (1979).

Nielsson, Haraldur. *Congrès International tenu á Varsovie en 1923.* Quoted in A. R. G. Owen, *Can We Explain the Poltergeist?* New York: Helix Press, 1964.

Ornstein, Robert. *The Psychology of Consciousness.* London: Cape, 1975.

Osty, Eugene. *Supernormal Faculties in Man.* London: Methuen, 1923.

Oswald, Ian. *Sleep.* Harmondsworth: Penguin, 1966.

Owen, A. R. G. *Can We Explain the Poltergeist?* New York: Helix Press, 1964.

Peterson, John M. "Left-Handedness: Differences Between Student Artists and Scientists." *Perceptual and Motor Skills* 48 (1979).

"Philip the Man-made Phantom." *Alpha,* May/June (1979).

Phylos the Tibetan. *A Dweller on Two Planets.* New York: Harper, 1974.

Pietsch, Paul. *Shufflebrain.* Boston: Houghton Mifflin, 1981.

Prescott, James. "Forebrain, Midbrain and Hindbrain Correlations." 1985.

———. "Phylogenetic and Ontogenetic Aspects of Human Affectional Development." In R. Gemme and C. C. Wheeler, eds., *Progress in Sexology.* New York: Plenum Press, 1977.

————. "Early Somatosensory Deprivation as an Ontogenetic Process in the Abnormal Development of the Brain and Behaviour." In I. E. Goldsmith and J. Moor-Jankowski, *Medical Primatology*. New York: Karger, 1971.

Prince, Morton. *The Dissociation of Personality*. Oxford: Oxford University Press, 1978.

Pringle, M. L. K. *11,000 Seven-Year-Olds*. London: Longmans, 1976.

Puharich, Andrija. *Uri*. London: W. H. Allen, 1974.

Raine, Kathleen. *Blake and the New Age*. London: Allen & Unwin, 1979.

Rees, W. Demi. "The Hallucinations of Widowhood." *British Medical Journal* 4 (1971).

Rhine, J. B., and Sara R. Feather. "The Study of Cases of Psi-Trailing in Animals." *Journal of Parapsychology* 26 (1962).

Roberts, Jane. *Psychic Politics*. Upper Saddle River, N.J.: Prentice Hall, 1976.

Roll, William G. *The Poltergeist*. Metuchen, N.J.: Scarecrow Press, 1976.

Rose, Ronald. *Living Magic*. New York: Rand McNally, 1956.

Roth, W. F., and F. H. Luton. "The Mental Health Programme in Tennessee." *American Journal of Psychiatry* 99 (1943).

Sackeim, H. A., et al. "Emotions Are Expressed More Intensely on the Left Side of the Face." *Science* 202 (1978).

Schatzman, Morton. *The Story of Ruth*. London: Duckworth, 1980.

"Schizophrenia: The Case for Viruses." *New Scientist*, 10 February (1983).

Schopenhauer, Arthur. *Parerga and Paralipomena*. Oxford: Oxford University Press, 1974.

Schreiber, Flora Rheta. *Sybil*. Harmondsworth, U.K.: Penguin. 1975.

Schurmacher, Emile. *Strange Unsolved Mysteries*. Cited in Colin Wilson, *The Occult*. London: Hodder, 1971.

Selfe, Lorna. *Nadia—A Case of Extraordinary Drawing Ability in an Autistic Child*. London: Academic Press, 1977.

Shackley, Myra. *Wild Men: Yeti, Sasquatch and the Neanderthal Enigma*. London: Thames & Hudson, 1983.

Shorter, Eric. "Raped by No One, but the Bruises Remain." *Daily Telegraph*, 1 October (1982).

Shuttle, Penelope, and Peter Redgrove. *The Wise Wound*. London: Goliancz, 1978.

Sidgwick, Eleanor. "Phantasms of the Living." *Proceedings*, Society for Psychical Research, vol. 33 (1922).

Sidis, Boris, and Simon Goodhart. *Multiple Personality.* New York: Greenwood Press, 1968.

Simon, Ted. "That Was No Lady, That's a Ghost." *The Times,* 3 January (1983).

Singer, Isaac Bashevis. *The Séance.* London: Cape, 1970.

Sizemore, Chris, and Elen Pittillo. *Eve.* London: Gollancz, 1978.

Sklair, Freda. Personal communication to the author.

Smith, Aaron. "Speech and Other Functions after Left (Dominant) Hemispherectomy." *Journal of Neurology, Neurosurgery and Psychiatry* 29 (1966).

Sperry, R. W. "The Great Cerebral Commissure." *Scientific American* 210 (1964).

Spiegl, Anni. *The Life and Death of Therese Neumann of Konnersreuth.* Susan Johnson, trans. Eichstatt, 1973.

"Spontaneous Hallucinations of the Sane." *Proceedings,* Society for Psychical Research, vol. 10 (1894).

Stevenson, Ian. *Twenty Cases Suggestive of Reincarnation.* Charlottesville, Va.: University of Virginia Press, 1974.

Sulloway, Frank J. *Freud, Biologist of the Mind.* New York: Basic Books, 1979.

Summers, Montague. *The History of Witchcraft and Demonology.* London: Routledge, 1973.

Summers, Montague (Sinistrari de Ameno). *Demonality or Incubi and Succubi.* London: Fortune Press, 1927.

Swedenborg, E. *Heaven and Hell.* London: Swedenborg Society, 1896.

Tarver, W. J. Letter. *New Scientist,* 24 October (1968).

Taylor, Gordon Rattray. *The Natural History of the Mind.* London: Secker & Warburg, 1979.

Teng, E. L., et al. "Handedness in a Chinese Population." *Science* 193 (1976).

Thigpen, Corbett H., and Hervey M. Cleckley. *The Three Faces of Eve.* New York: McGraw Hill, 1957.

Thurston, Gavin. "Preternatural Combustion of the Human Body." *Medico-Legal Journal* 29 (1961).

Thurston, H. *Ghosts and Poltergeists.* London: Burns Oates, 1953.

Tomas, Andrew. *We Are Not the First.* London: Sphere, 1972.

Twigg, Ena, and R. H. Brod. *Ena Twigg, Medium.* London: W. H. Allen, 1973.

Underwood, Peter. *Dictionary of the Supernatural.* London: Harrap, 1978.

Usher, Shaun. "Can This Boy Be Ten Different People?" *Daily Mail,* 24 October (1978).

Wallace, Marjorie. "The Day They Gave This Man His Memory Back." *Sunday Times,* 24 April (1983).

Weitzenhoffer, A. M. *Hypnotism.* New York: Wiley, 1963.

Wheeler, W. M., et al. "The Internal Structure of the MMPI." *Journal of Consulting Psychology* 15 (1951).

Wieschoff, Heinz A. "Concepts of Right and Left in African Cultures." In Rodney Needham, *Left and Right.* Chicago: University of Chicago Press, 1973.

Williams, Mary. "The Poltergeist Man." *Journal of Analytical Psychology* 8 (1963).

Willoughby-Meade, Gerald. *Chinese Ghouls and Goblins.* London: Constable, 1928.

Wilson, Ian. *Mind Out Of Time?* London: Gollancz, 1981.

Woolf, Leonard. *Beginning Again.* London: Harrap, 1964.

Wright, Pearce. "The No-Brain Genius May Be on Its Way." *The Times,* 30 December (1980).

Yeats, W. B. *Essays and Introductions.* London: Macmillan, 1961.

Young, H. B., and R. Knapp. "Personality Characteristics of Converted Left-Handers." *Perceptual and Motor Skills* 23 (1965).

INDEX